# PUBLISHER'S NOTE

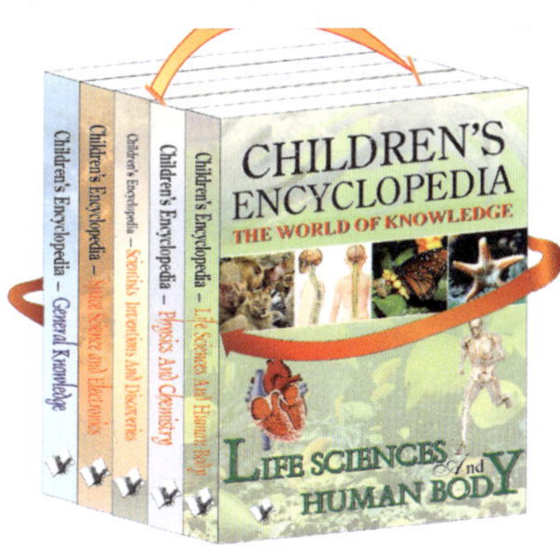


**V&S Publishers** — Leading Publisher of Children and Academic Books in India for over a decade, is glad to announce the launch of a unique, fully *coloured set of five books* under the head, ***Children's Encyclopedia – The World of Knowledge.*** The set of 5 books namely – ***Life Sciences and the Human Body, Physics and Chemistry, Space Science and Electronics, Scientists and Inventions*** and ***General Knowledge*** has been especially developed keeping in mind the students and children of all age groups, particularly from 6 to 14 years of age. Our main aim is to arouse interest and solve queries of the school children regarding various and diverse topics of Science and help them master the subject thoroughly. After the resounding success of 71 Science Trailblazing Series, we present you with this new arrival of ours.

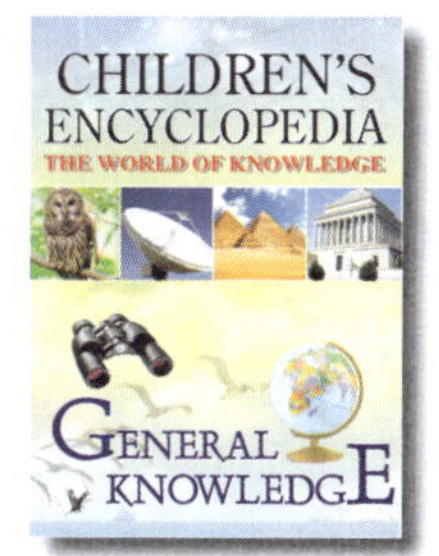


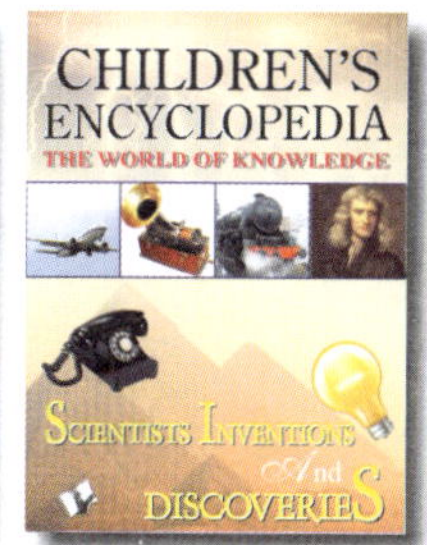


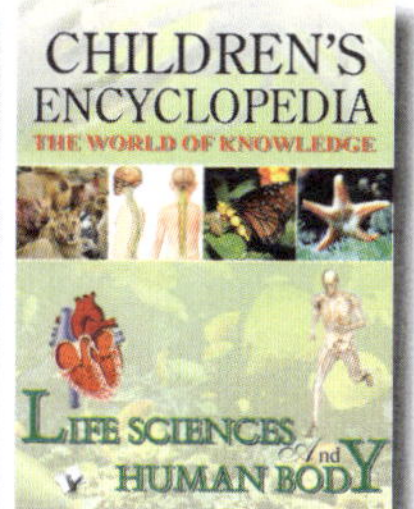


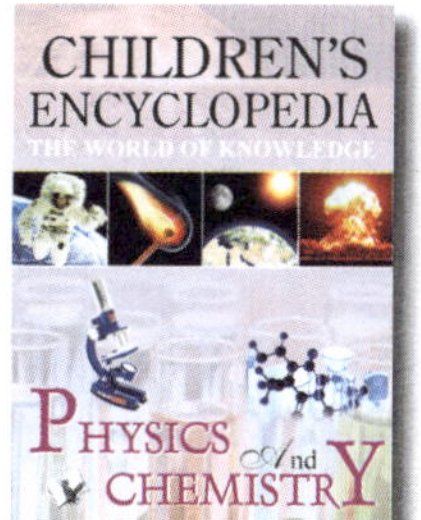


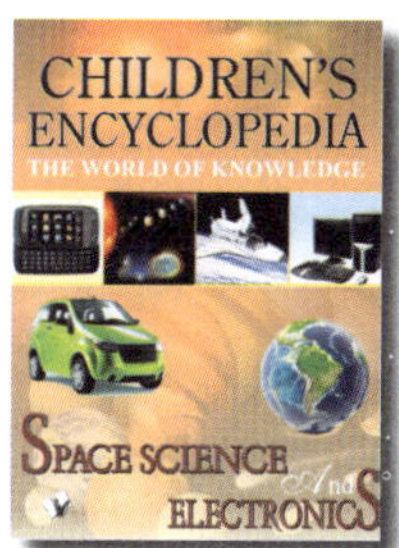


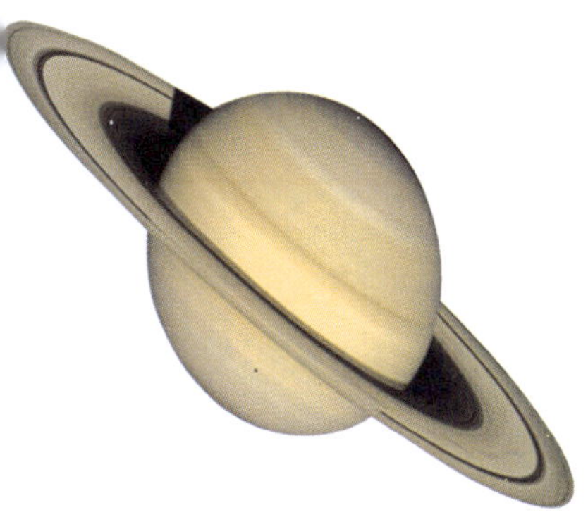

In the book, ***Space Science and Electronics,*** the author has broadly dealt with some interesting and fascinating Scientific facts in the first part (Part-I) like *The Universe, The Stars, The Solar System, The Sun, The Moons, The Meteorites, The Comets*, etc. The second part (Part-II), on the other hand, focusses mainly on the *Ancient, Medieval and Modern Means of Transportation, Types of Transportation, The Roadways, The Railways, The Airways and The Waterways, Supersonic Means of Transportation, Transportation in Armed Forces* and so on…

Each chapter is followed by a section called **Quick Facts** that contains a set of interesting and fascinating facts about the topics already discussed in the chapter. There are also **Exercises** compiled at the end of the book followed by a **Glossary** of difficult words and scientific terms to make the book complete and comprehensive.

*Though our aim is to be flawless, but errors might have crept in inadvertently. So we request our esteemed readers to read the book thoroughly and offer valuable suggestions wherever necessary to improve and enhance the quality of the book. Hope it interests you all and serves its purpose well.*

# CONTENTS

## PART-I SPACE SCIENCE

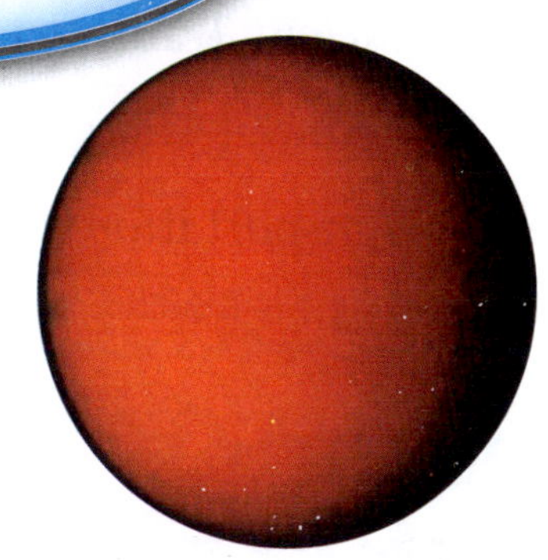

### PART- I SPACE



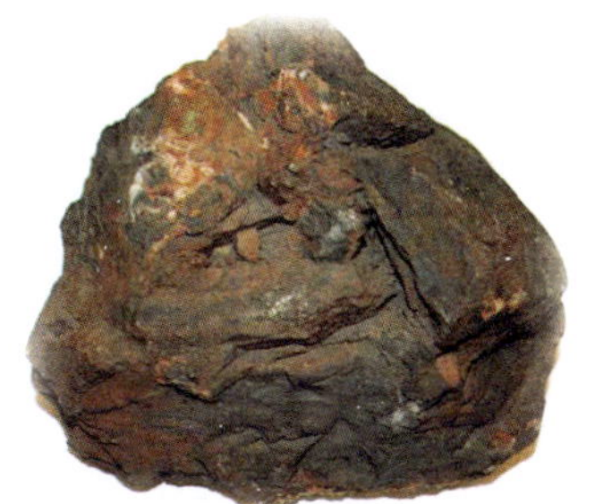



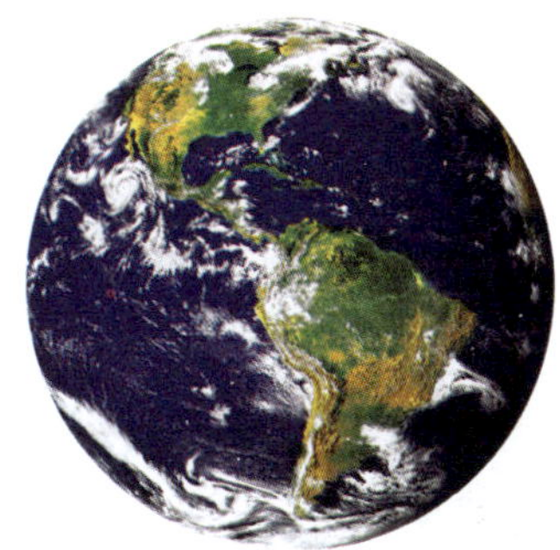

### PART- II THE EARTH



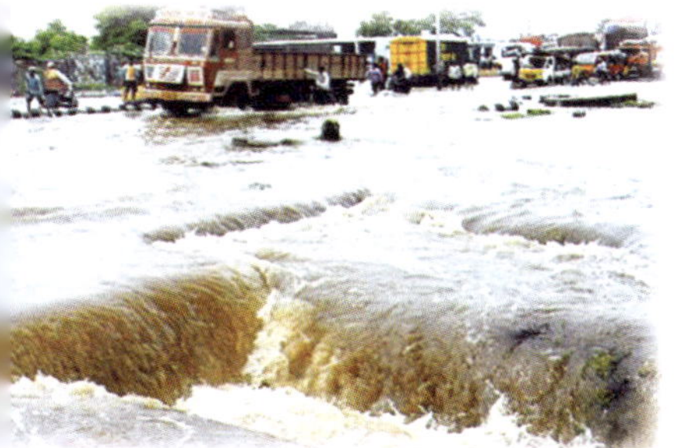

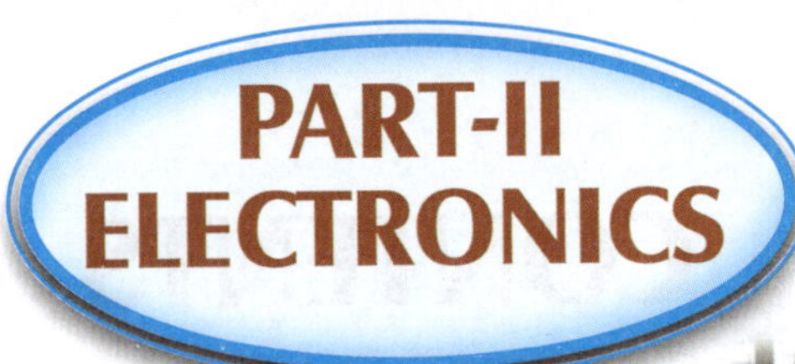


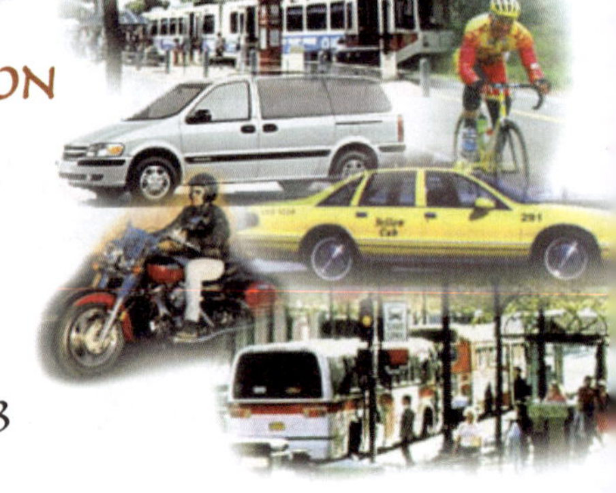

## PART-I ELECTRONICS AND TRANSPORTATION



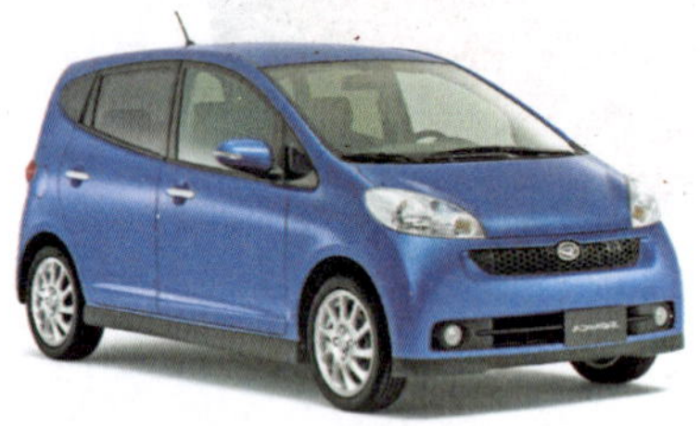



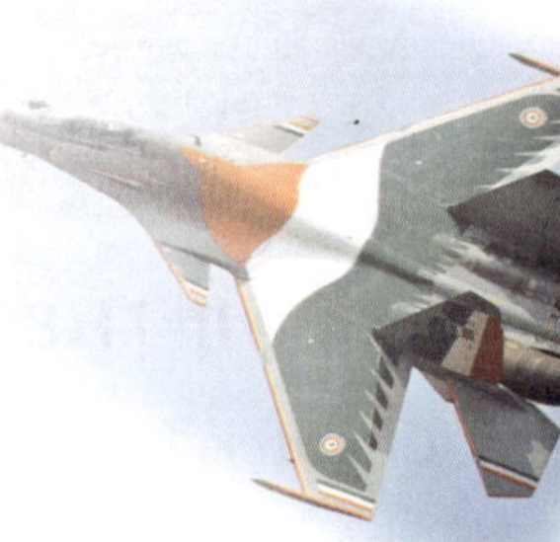

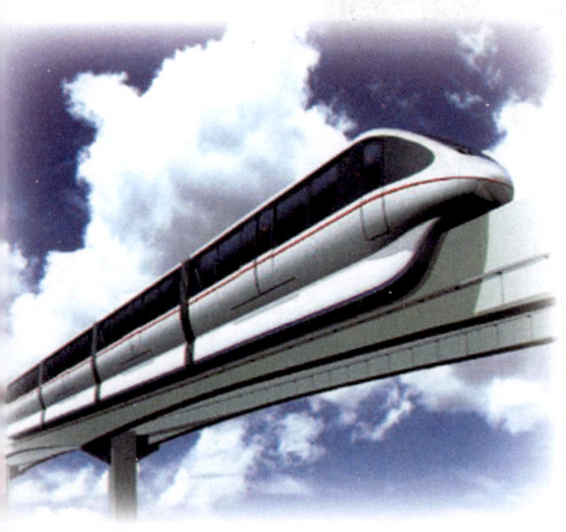

## PART-II ELECTRONICS AND COMMUNICATIONS



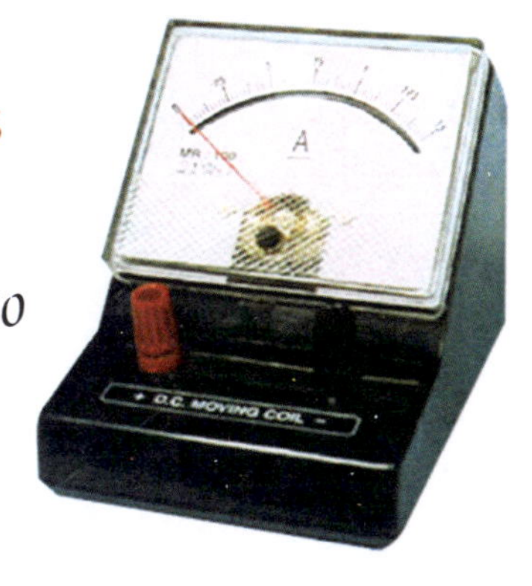


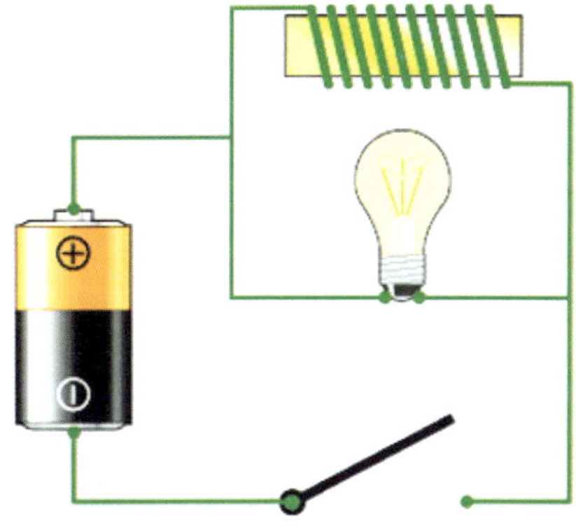



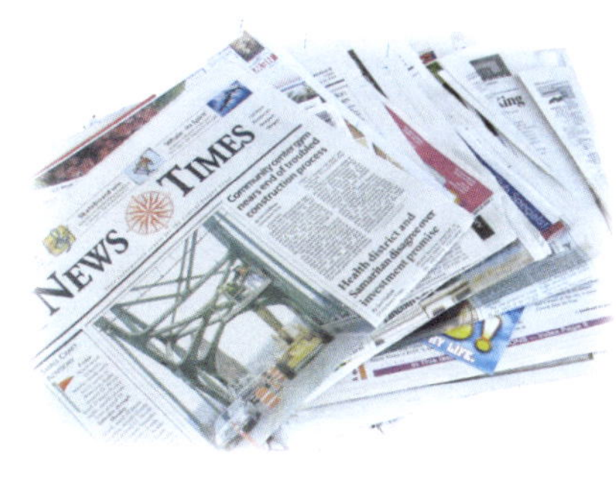


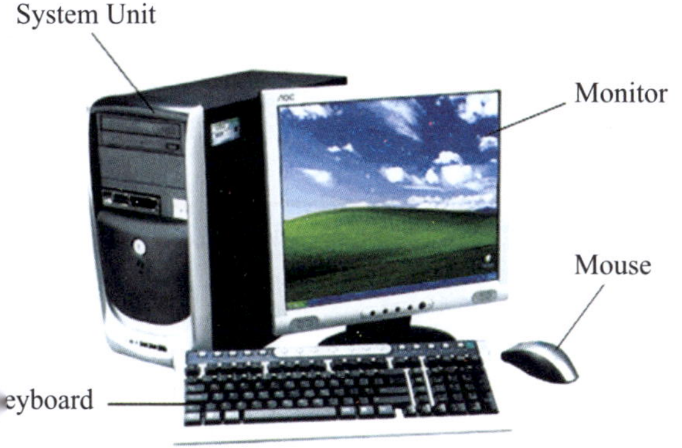

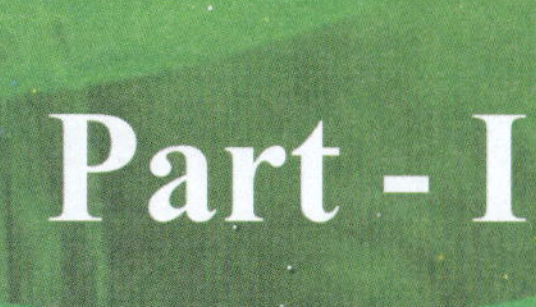


# SPACE

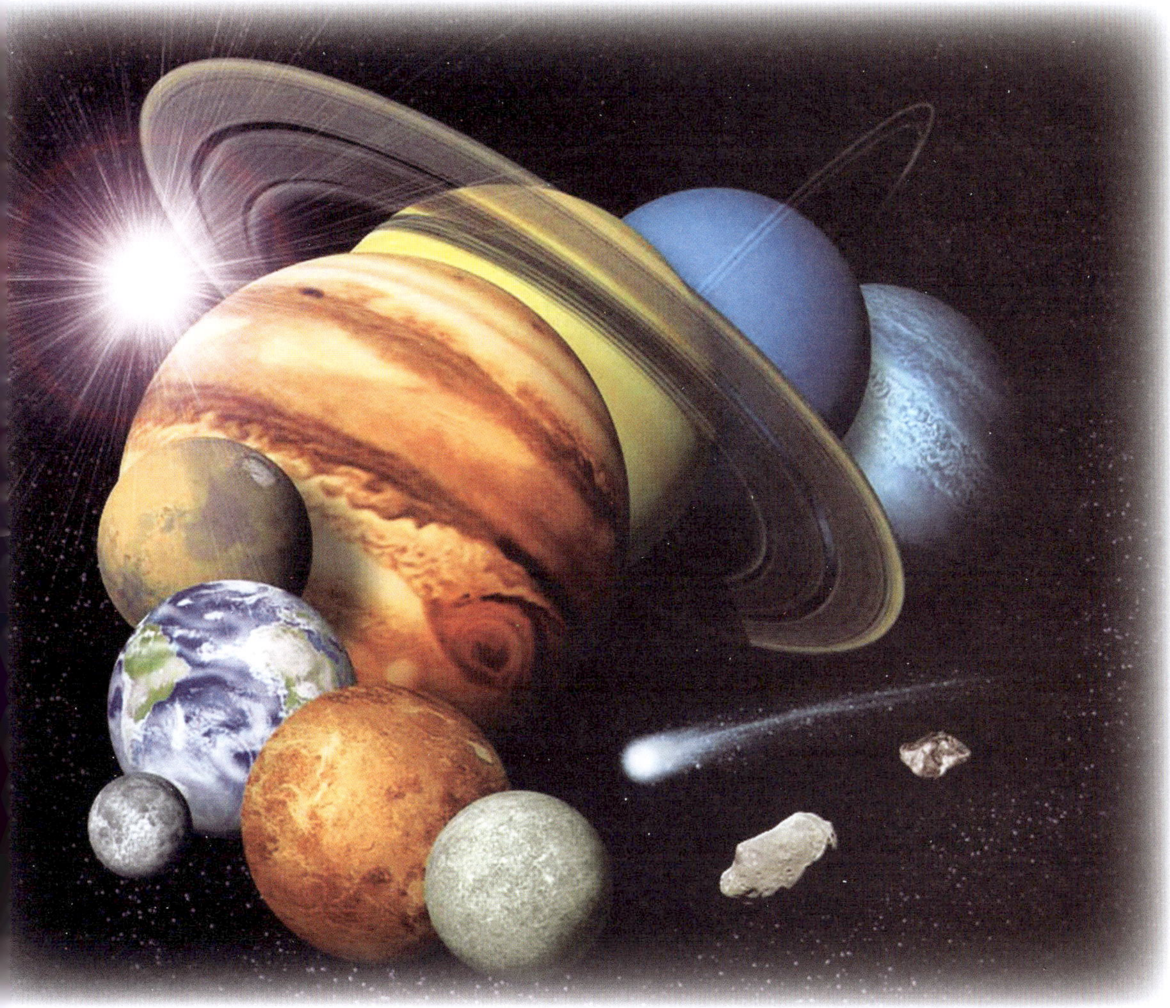

# Chapter - 1

# THE UNIVERSE

About 13.7 billion years ago, the Universe was formed in a massive explosion called the **Big Bang**. The Universe consists of everything that exists:

- Matter
- Space
- Time
- Energy

All of these are parts of the Universe.

Energy is of various types: *light, sound, motion* and even *heat*. Matter, on the other hand, can easily be seen with the naked eye. All the objects around us are made up of matter.

Even today, the Universe continues to *expand, cool* and *change*. This phenomenon was discovered by the American astronomer, **Vesto Slipher** in 1910.

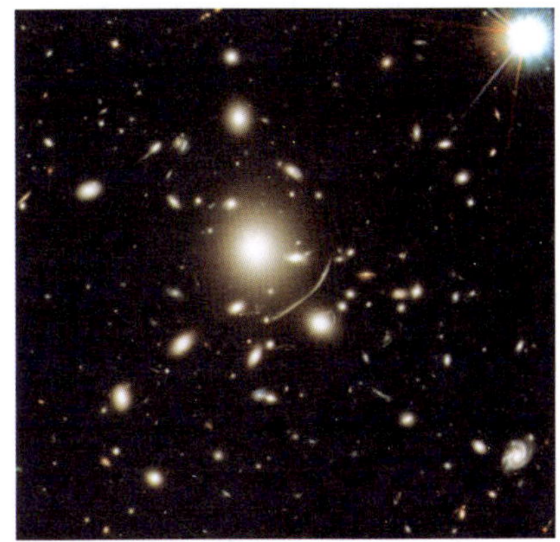

*Space*

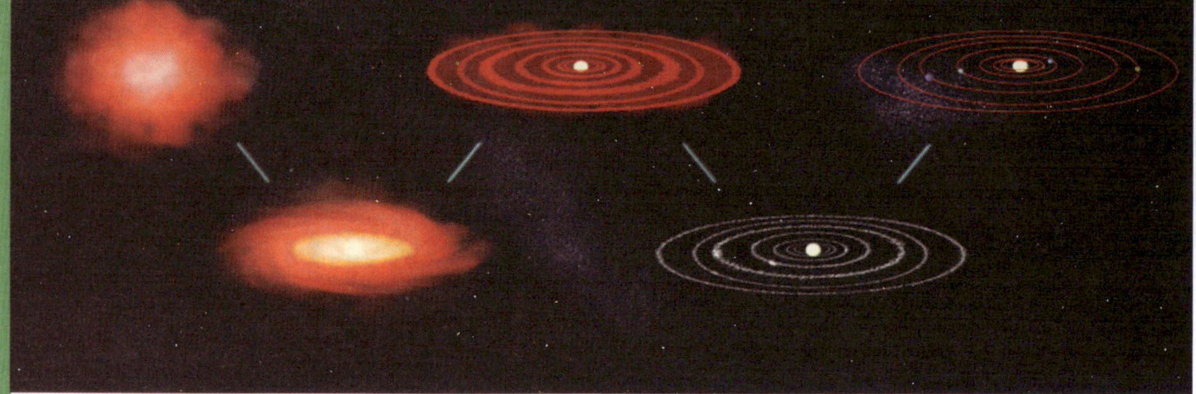

**Big Bang** → 200 million years after Big Bang → **Formation of Stars** → 500 million years after the Big Bang → **Formation of Galaxies** → 1 billion years after Big Bang → **Galaxies with different shapes exist in the Universe** → 9 billion years after Big Bang → Formation of our Solar System

## Big Bang

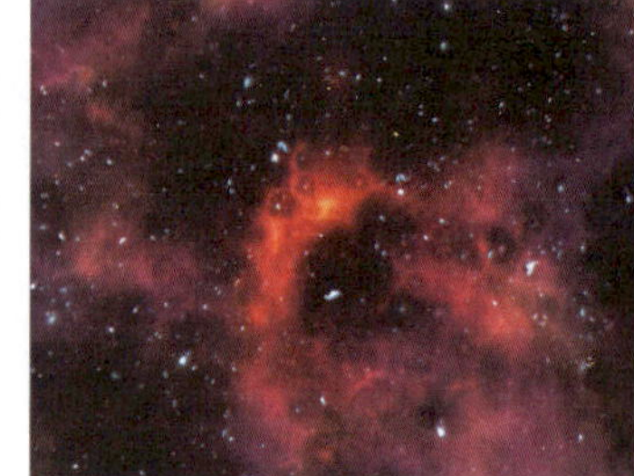

The Big Bang

The Big Bang is the way the Universe began. It was not a sound, but an *enormous explosion* in which a large amount of energy was produced, causing the space to suddenly expand. This energy turned into matter on its own, forming the Universe. Astronomers (scientists who study various bodies in the Universe) can tell that the Big Bang took place and some of that energy still exists and continues to fill the Universe with energy even today. This energy is known as the *Cosmic Microwave Background Radiation*.

Even though astronomers today have various explanations as to how the Universe developed from the Big Bang, they do not know what caused the Big Bang.

## Galaxies

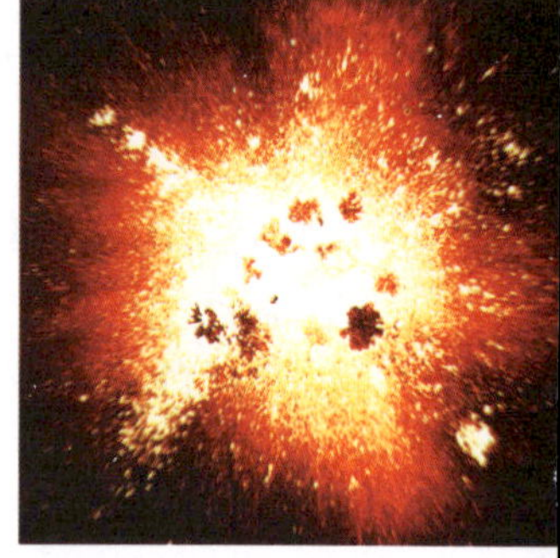

Galaxies

About one billion years after the Big Bang, galaxies were formed in the Universe. *A galaxy is a very large group of stars which are held together by gravity* (a force that causes objects to fall on the ground).

According to a scientific research, there are about 100–125 billion galaxies in the Universe. Each galaxy has more than 1,00,000 million stars.

*Different galaxies have different shapes.* Five basic shapes have been discovered till today. These are:

i. Elliptical Galaxy
ii. Lenticular or Lens-shaped Galaxy
iii. Spiral Galaxy
iv. Barred Spiral Galaxy
v. Irregular Galaxy

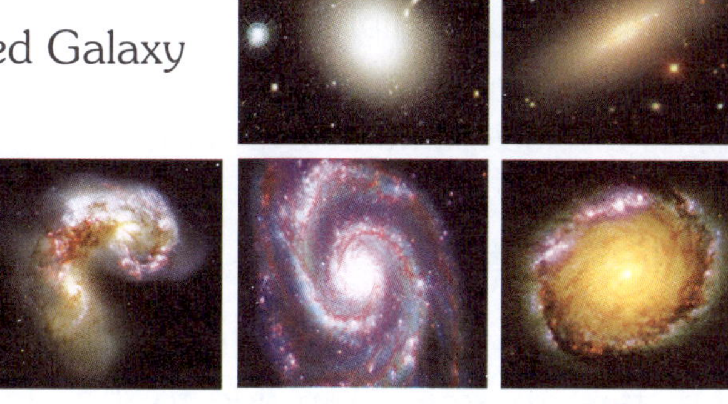

*Different Galaxies*

## The Milky Way

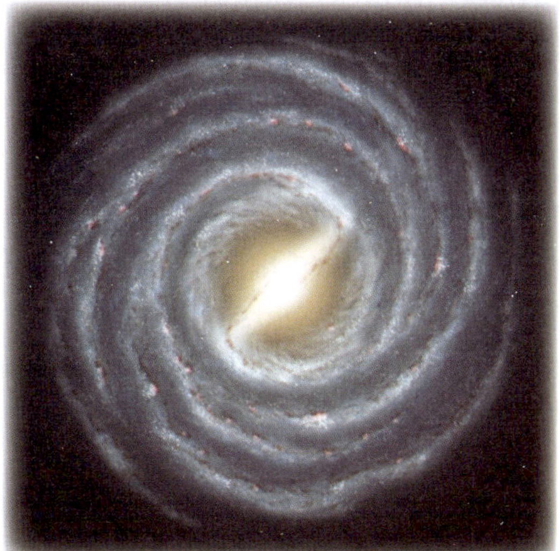

*The Milky Way*

The galaxy we live in is called the *Milky Way*. It was formed about one billion years after the Big Bang, at the same time as all the other galaxies. The Sun, the other Planets, the Stars and everything else are all a part of the Milky Way. According to astronomers, the Milky Way is a *spiral galaxy*.

The Milky Way rotates on its axis (an imaginary line through the middle of anything), faster at the centre than at the edges. The centre completes one rotation on its axis in about 50,000 years. The sun and its neighbouring stars revolve around the centre of the galaxy in their orbits at an average speed of 250 kilometres per second.

## Andromeda Galaxy

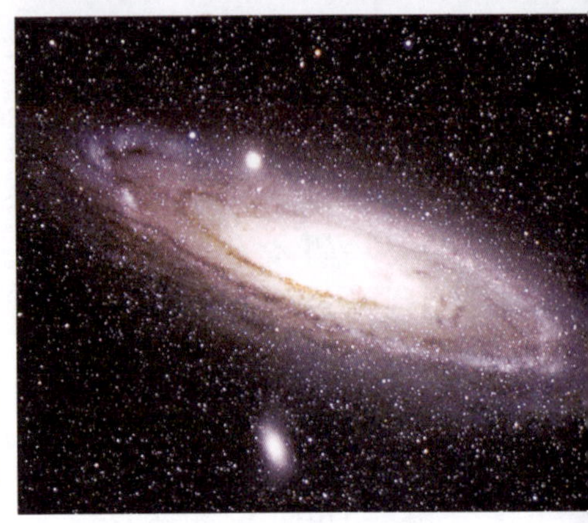

*Andromeda Galaxy*

Andromeda is the *closest galaxy to the Milky Way*. It is about *2.9 million light years away from the Earth*, which means that it will take us around 2.2 million years to get there, that also if we are travelling at the speed of light. This spiral-shaped galaxy can be seen from the earth without using any scientific instrument.

## Edge of the Universe

Even though, early astronomers believed that somewhere beyond the stars, there was an end to the Universe, but studies have now proved that no matter how fast and how far you travel, *there is no end to the Universe.*

## Size of the Universe

Even though, no study or research has ever been able to determine the actual size of the Universe, we know that the Universe is at least *90 billion light years across*. This has been determined by calculating the distance between the Earth and the most distant objects that can be seen.

## End of the Universe

There are many theories about how the Universe will come to an end. Out of these, most scientists believe that the Universe will either continue to expand and cool, till it eventually becomes dark and dead or all the objects that make up the Universe, such as galaxies, stars, etc., will rip themselves apart. It could also happen that the Universe stops expanding and then crashes into itself.

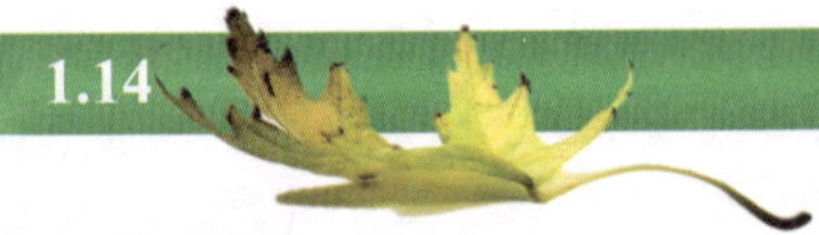

## Quick Facts

- The name Big Bang was given by famous English astronomer, Fred Hoyle, who surprisingly did not believe in the theory himself. He was just making fun, but the name struck.
- Physicist Albert Einstein gave the mathematical model of the Universe in 1917. This model is still used today. The Big Bang Theory was suggested ten years later by Belgian astronomer Georges Lemaître.
- The Universe is also known as the Cosmos. Also, the study of the whole Universe is known as Cosmology.
- There are around 200 to 400 billion stars in the Milky Way.

Chapter - 2

# THE STARS

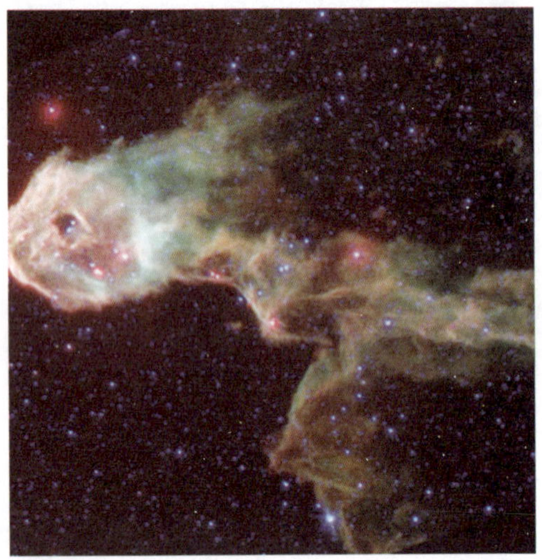

Stars are nothing but huge balls made of hot, luminous gases, which spin continuously. No two stars are the same. Each star has a specific temperature, colour, brightness, size and mass. These characteristics of the star change over a period of time, and hence, the star evolves from one stage of its life to another.

The life of a star depends on the amount of gas it is made up from, which is called the *mass*. Not only the lifespan, but also the characteristics of a star depends on its mass.

## Life of a Star

Stars are born inside thick clouds of hydrogen gas in space called the *nebulae*. Clusters within the hydrogen clouds collapse inwards and are pulled together by gravity. They keep getting packed together and thus, keep becoming hotter.

## Nebulae

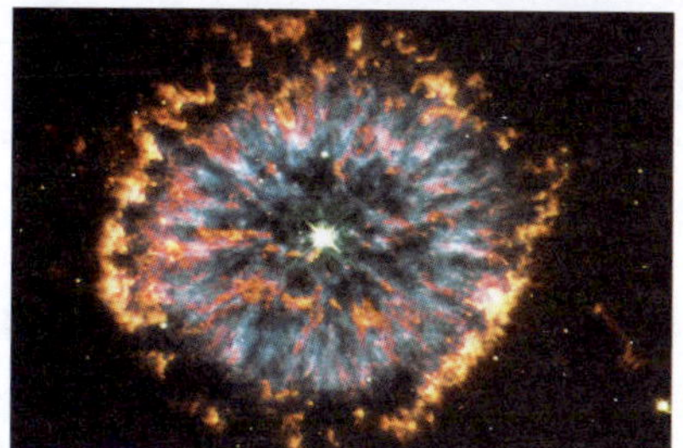
Nebulae

Gas, along with little knots of dust are pulled inside the nebulae due to gravity. Each one of these could become stars as gravity squeezes it tightly and it becomes hotter.

## Red Giants

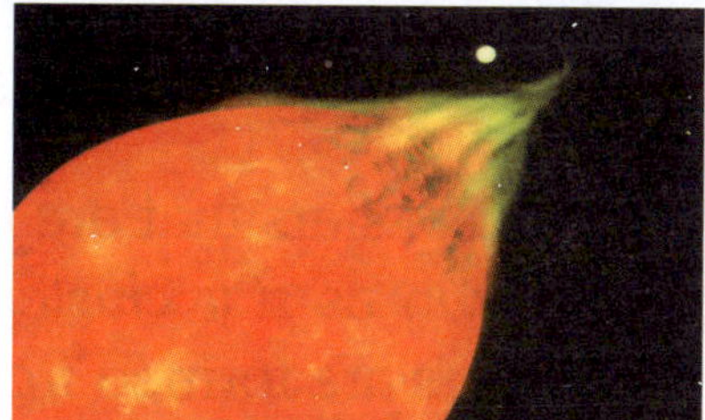
Red Giants

Stars are made up of *hydrogen gas*. Till the time they have hydrogen, they burn, after which they start to burn out. After this, they expand and become a *red giant star*.

## White Dwarfs

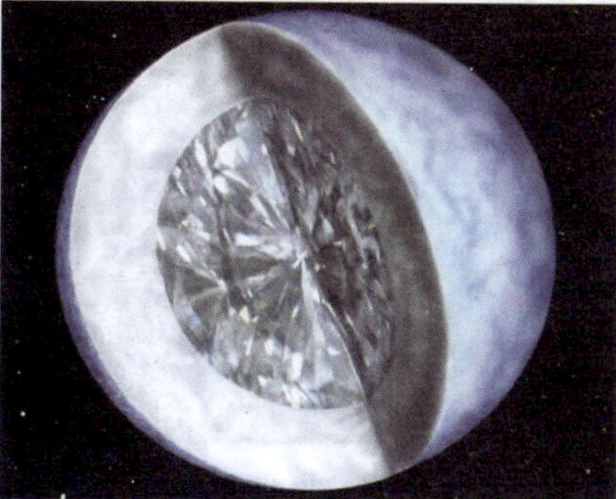
White Dwarfs

After some time, the outer layers of the stars are thrown into space. The only thing left is the cooling core. This is called a *white dwarf*. These white dwarfs are no bigger than the earth.

## Supernova

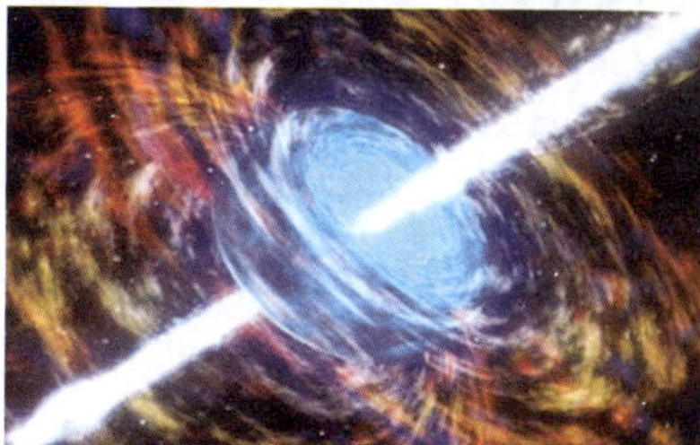
Supernova

The life of a massive star generally comes to an end with a huge *supernova explosion*.

## Remnants

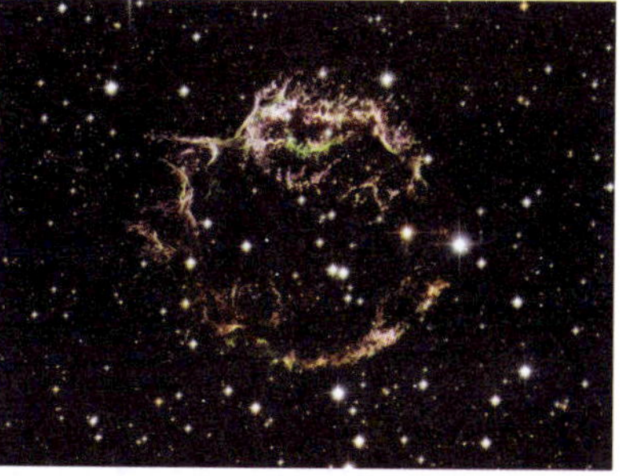
Remnants

A star's fragments or parts can remain in the space and continue to glow for hundreds of years.

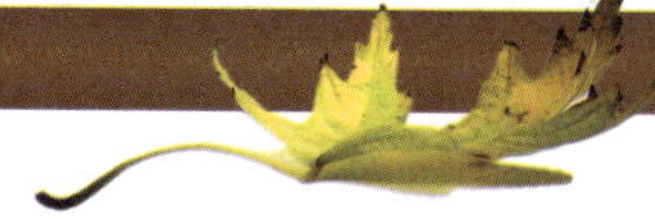

## Stars in Motion

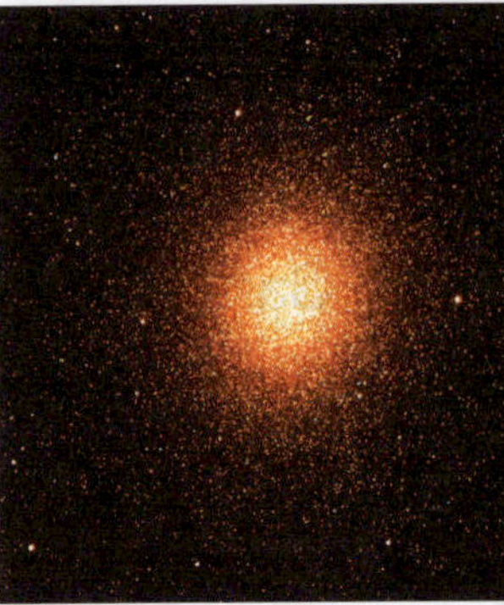

Even though stars seem to move at night, this is not true. It is not the stars, but the earth that moves beneath the stars, which are in space.

## Types of Star Clusters

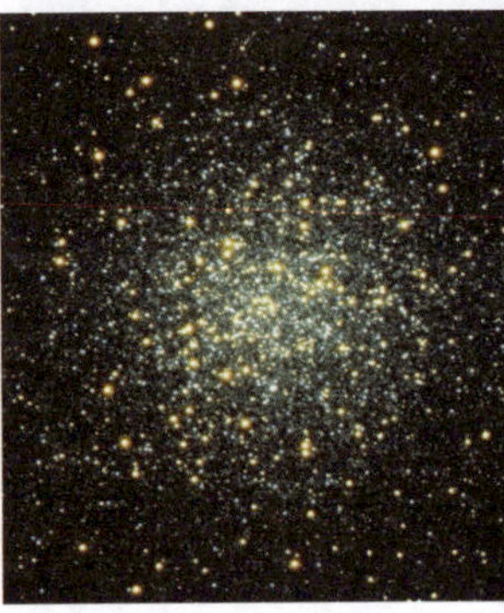

A group of stars that are close to each other in space are known as *star clusters*. This usually happens as these stars are formed from the same cloud.

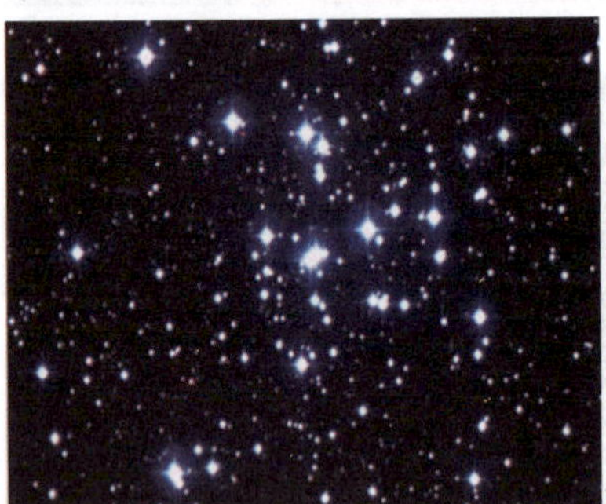

Clusters that are round in shape and have many stars packed closely together, are called *globular clusters*. On the other hand, clusters which have fewer and more spread out stars, are called *open clusters*.

## Biggest Star Found

Till date, the biggest star found by astronomers is called **VY Canis Majoris**. It is about 1,800 to 2,100 times the diameter (the length of a line that cuts across the centre of a circular object from one end to the other) of the sun, which means that a billion objects, the size of the sun, can fit into it. It is also extremely bright, i.e., many thousands of times brighter than the sun. It does not look bright during the night as it is about 5,000 light years away from us.

## Constellations

*Constellations are patterns of stars in the sky*. They were first used about *4,000 years ago*. Constellations are generally named either after a mythological creature or person, or after an object. Around

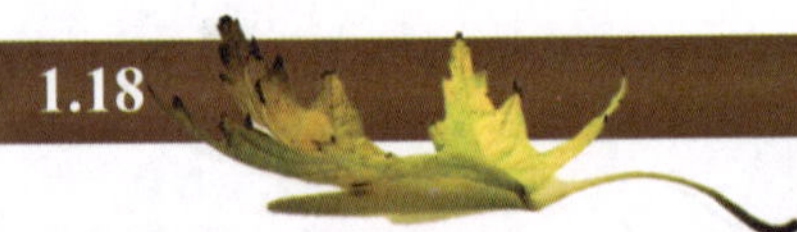

*88 constellations* have been identified in the sky till date. These help stargazers (people who study stars as an astronomer) find their way and navigate the sky.

The following are some of the popularly known constellations:

1. Gemini

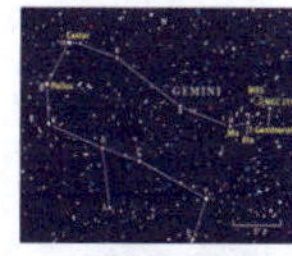

2. Taurus

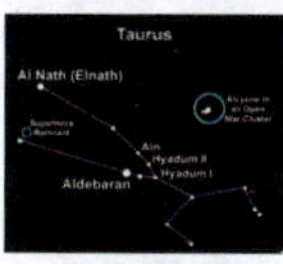


3. Canis Minor and Major

4. Monoceros

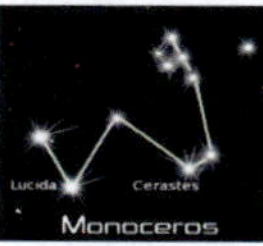


5. Orion

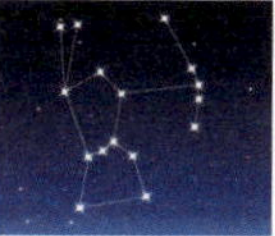

6. Eridanus

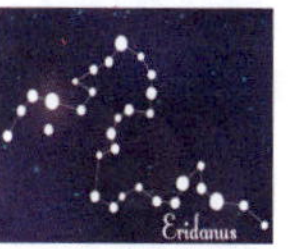


7. Puppis

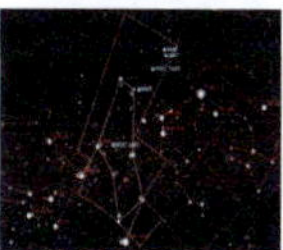

8. Lepus

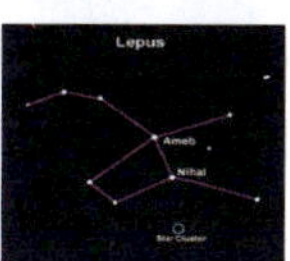

## Quick Facts

- We can see about 2,000 stars in the sky on a clear, dark night.
- A star is a colossal, glowing ball of plasma and the star that is nearest to the earth is the Sun.
- Stars, including the Sun, have spots on their surfaces – sometimes enormous ones. Spots are cooler areas. They are caused by powerful magnetic fields.
- Hydrogen is the primary building block of stars.
- Stars may occur in many sizes, which are classified in a range from dwarfs to super giants. Super giants may have radii a thousand times larger than that of our own Sun.
- The colour of Stars can range from red to white to blue. Red is the coolest colour; that's a star with less than 3,500 Kelvin temperature. Stars like the Sun are yellowish white and have an average temperature of around 6,000 Kelvin. The hottest stars are blue, which correspond to surface temperatures above 12,000 Kelvin.

# Chapter - 3

# THE SOLAR SYSTEM

The Solar System is a small part of the space. It consists of the Sun, the Eight Planets, and innumerable other smaller objects.

In the beginning, the Solar System was nothing but a *huge cloud of dust and gas*. When it collapsed, pulled together by its gravity, a

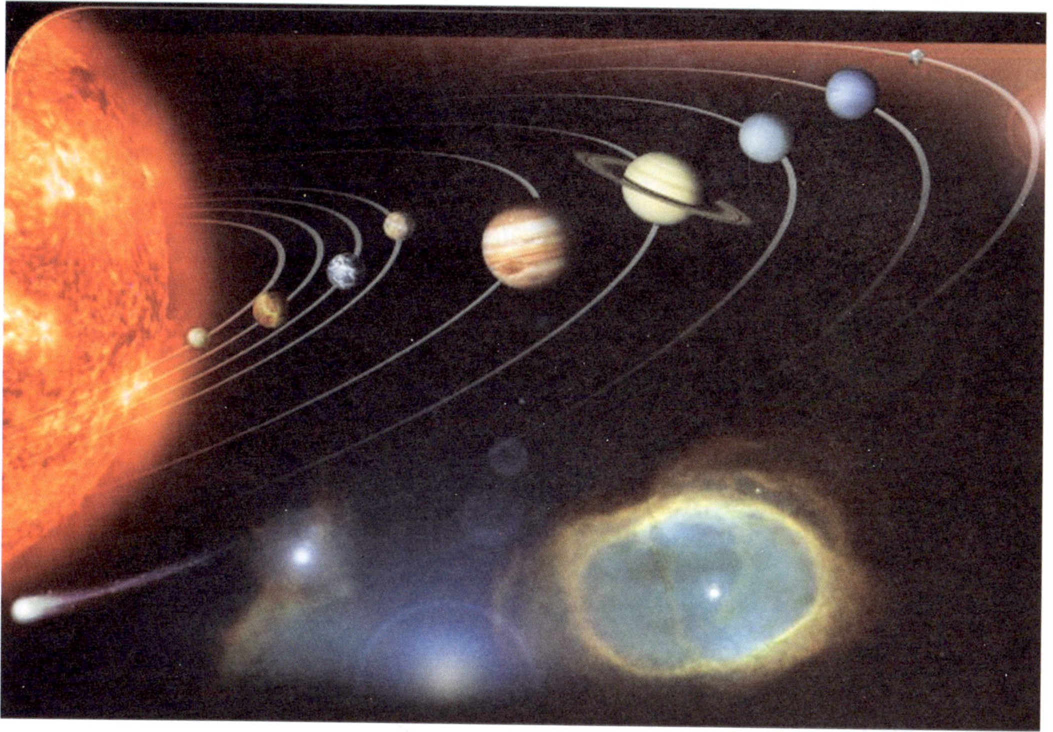

*Solar System*

part of it became very dense and hot, turning into the Sun. All the materials that were left settled into a spinning disc around the Sun, where the planets and other objects that make up the Solar System formed.

The Solar System is enormous. Our Earth is just a tiny part of it. The closest natural object to the Earth is the Moon. As it orbits the earth, its distance from the earth also keeps on changing. At its furthest point, it is about 4,05,696 kilometres (2,52,088 miles) from the earth, while at its closest point, it is around 3,63,104 kilometres (2,25,622 miles) from the earth. Neptune is the farthest planet in our Solar System and its distance is about 4.5 billion kilometres (2.8 billion miles) from the sun.

The Solar System is not static and is constantly changing. Other than forming planets, some of the materials that formed the Solar System remained as *asteroids*, *comets*, and *other small bodies*. Till about 3.8 billion years ago, these objects quite often collided with the planets, due to which *craters* were formed. Even though the number of such collisions has drastically reduced, they still happen.

## Planets

There are **eight planets** in the *Solar System*:

(i) Mercury

(ii) Venus

(iii) Earth

(iv) Mars

(v) Jupiter

(vi) Saturn

(vii) Uranus

(viii) Neptune

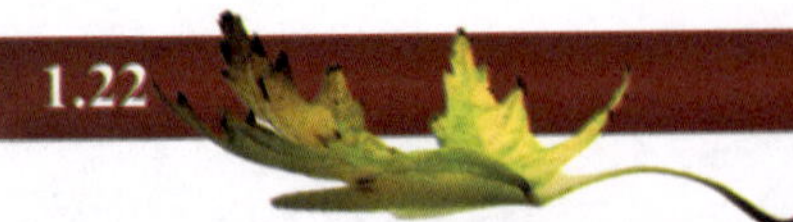

*Mercury is the closest to the sun, while Neptune is the farthest.* All the planets orbit the sun in the same direction. *Mercury, Venus, Earth and Mars* are completely made up of rocks while *Jupiter, Saturn, Uranus* and *Neptune* are made up of various gases. Due to this, they are also known as gas planets. As the planets go farther away from the sun, the time they take to orbit or move around the sun once, also increases. This happens because their distance from the sun increases. If we calculate in terms of the days on the planet, Earth, *Mercury only takes 88 days to complete one round around the sun, while Neptune takes about 64.8 years.*

## Mercury

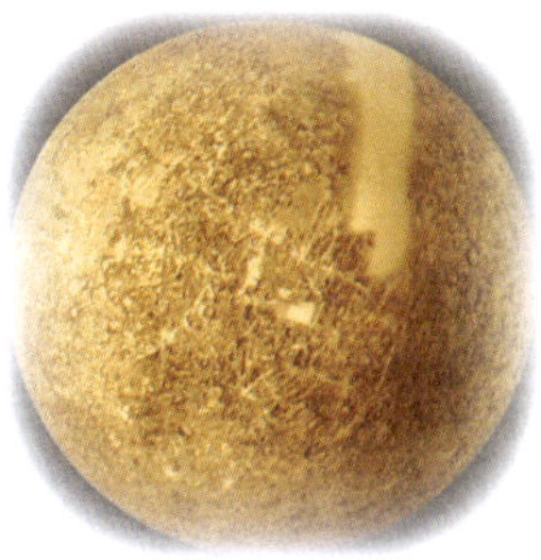

*Mercury*

Made up of rocks and covered with innumerable impact craters, Mercury is a **dry planet**. It is the smallest planet of our Solar System. As it is the closest to the sun, it has the widest temperature range. Mercury is baking hot during the day, but freezing cold at night. Even though, it is difficult to see it without a telescope, (an instrument with lenses in it that help make distant objects look nearer) during the day due to its nearness to the sun and its small size, *Mercury can be easily spotted before sunrise or after sunset.*

| Data | Mercury |
|---|---|
| Diameter | 4,875 km<br>(3,029 miles) |
| Average distance from the sun | 57.9 million km<br>(36 million miles) |
| Rotation period | 58.6 days |
| Orbital period | 88 days |

## Venus

Venus is the second planet from the sun. It is not only the hottest, but also the brightest planet in the Solar System. It is made up of rocks and is always surrounded by a thick cloud that traps heat and makes it a *gloomy planet*.

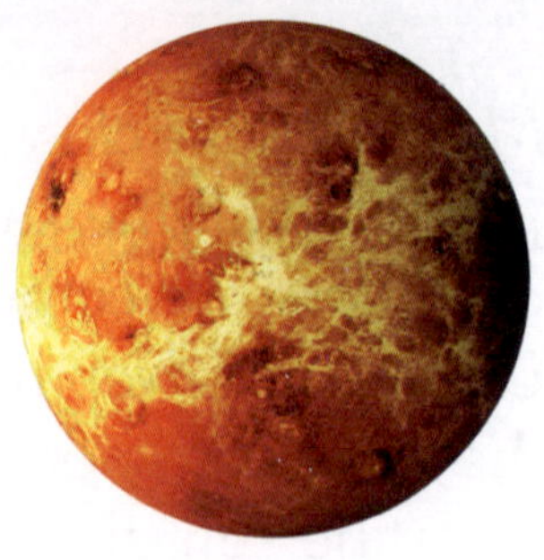

*Venus*

| Data | Venus |
|---|---|
| Diameter | 12,104 km (7,521 miles) |
| Average distance from the sun | 108.2 million km (67.2 million miles) |
| Rotation period | 243 days |
| Orbital period | 224.7 days |

## Earth

Out of the eight planets in our Solar System, the *Earth is the only planet that has life and liquid water*. Third from the sun, the Earth is the largest planet that is made of rocks. The surface of the Earth continues to change due to the movements in its crust. The Earth also has one natural satellite, called the Moon.

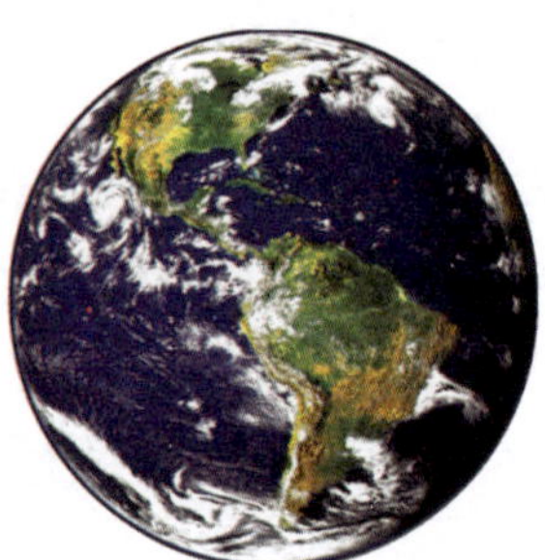

*Earth*

| Data | Earth |
|---|---|
| Diameter | 12,756 km (7,928 miles) |
| Average distance from the sun | 149.6 million km (93 million miles) |
| Rotation period | 23.93 hours |
| Orbital period | 365.26 days |

## Mars

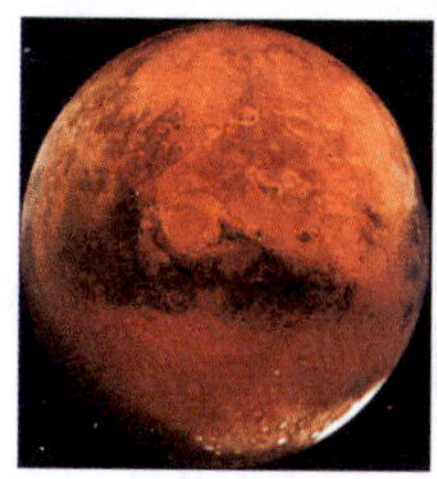

Mars

Mars is also known as the **red planet**. Out of all the rocky planets, it is the farthest from the sun and is extremely dry and cold. Its surface contains *deep canyons*, *frozen deserts*, *giant volcanoes* and *polar ice caps*. These have all been formed in the past. It also has *two moons*.

| Data | Mars |
|---|---|
| Diameter | 6,780 km<br>(4,213 miles) |
| Average distance from the sun | 227.9 million km<br>(141.6 million miles) |
| Rotation period | 24.62 hours |
| Orbital period | 687 days |

## Jupiter

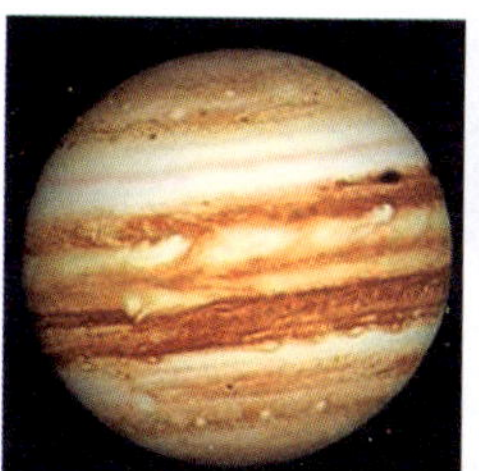

Jupiter

Jupiter is the *largest planet in our Solar System*. Not only is it the largest planet, but it also *spins the fastest*, completing one rotation on its own axis in less than 10 Earth hours. It is mostly made up of *helium* and *hydrogen*, but has a central *rocky core*. Jupiter has a *ring around* it, which is very thin and faint. It also has a large *family of moons*.

| Data | Jupiter |
|---|---|
| Diameter | 1,42,984 km<br>(88,846 miles) |
| Average distance from the sun | 778.3 million km<br>(483.6 million miles) |
| Rotation period | 9.93 hours |
| Orbital period | 11.86 years |

## Saturn

Saturn is the *second largest planet* in the Solar System. It is *pale yellow in colour* and is mainly made up of helium and hydrogen. Saturn also has a rocky core. It has a large family of moons and its distinctive feature is that it has a *ring system* which is made of innumerable pieces of dirty water and ice.

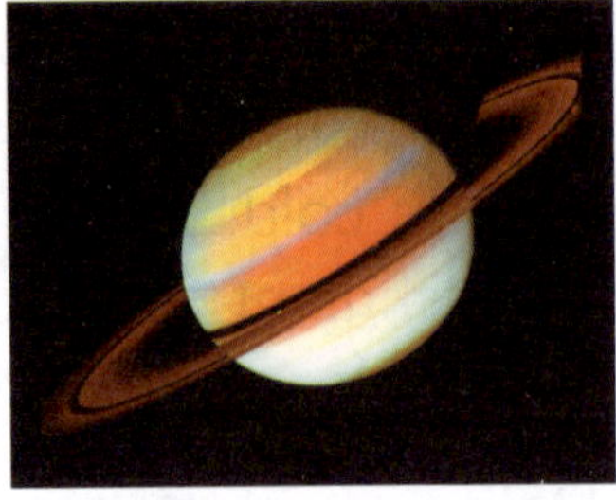

*Saturn*

| Data | Saturn |
|---|---|
| Diameter | 1,20,536 km (74,898 miles) |
| Average distance from the sun | 1,431 million km (889.8 million miles) |
| Rotation period | 10.65 hours |
| Orbital period | 29.37 years |

## Uranus

Uranus is the *seventh planet from the sun*. Its distance is nineteen times the distance of the sun from the earth. It is extremely cold and has a sparse ring system which encircles its equator (an imaginary line that cuts through the centre of the earth). It is an almost *featureless system* bounded by a *layer of haze*. As Uranus is tilted on its side, it appears as if its rings and moons orbit it from top to bottom.

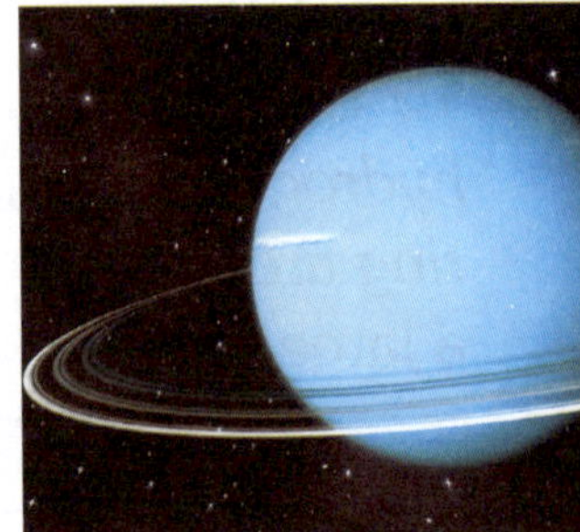

*Uranus*

| Data | Uranus |
|---|---|
| Diameter | 51,118 km (31,763 miles) |

| Average distance from the sun | 2,877 million km (1,788 million miles) |
|---|---|
| Rotation period | 17.24 hours |
| Orbital period | 84.1 years |

## Neptune

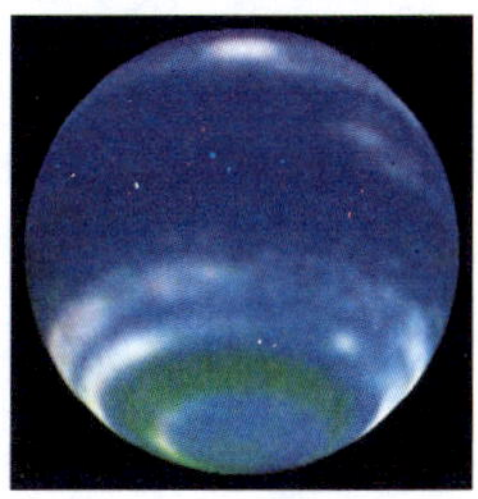
Neptune

Out of the eight planets in our Solar System, the **Neptune is the farthest**. It is also the windiest and the coldest. Its atmosphere consists of hydrogen-rich gas and the planet itself is basically made up of ammonia, methane and water ices. Neptune also has an extremely thin ring system and a large family of moons.

| Data | Neptune |
|---|---|
| Diameter | 51,118 km (30,775 miles) |
| Average distance from the sun | 4,498 million km (2,795 million miles) |
| Rotation period | 16.11 hours |
| Orbital period | 164.9 years |

## Dwarf Planets

Dwarf planets are small, roundish objects in the Solar System. Like all other objects in the Solar System, they also orbit the sun. Till date, **four dwarf planets** have been discovered. These are:

- Ceres
- Eris
- Pluto
- Makemake

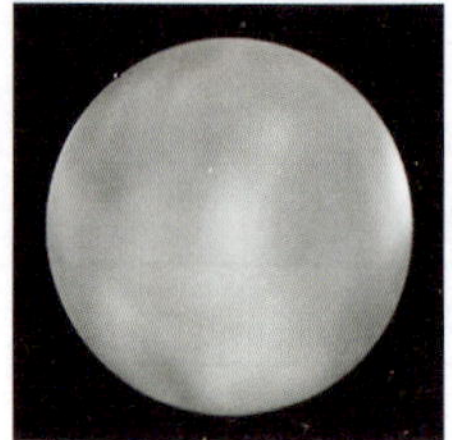 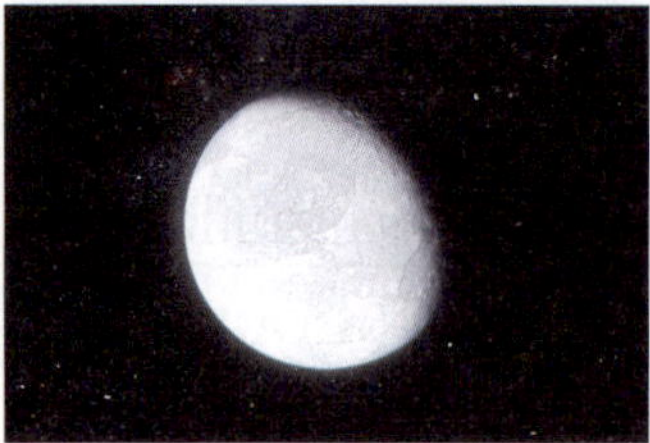 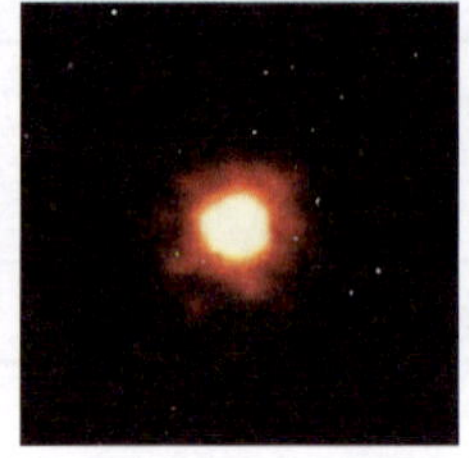 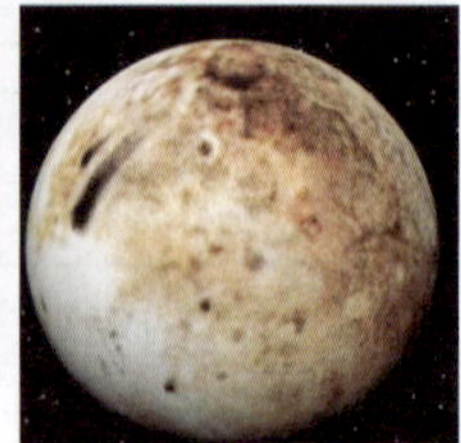

While Ceres orbits between Jupiter and Mars, within the Main Belt of asteroids, Pluto and Eris orbit beyond Neptune as part of the Kuiper Belt. The Kuiper Belt is a belt made of ice and rocky objects.

## Quick Facts

- **The Sun contains about 99.86% of the mass in the Solar System. It is about 73% hydrogen, so most of the matter in the Solar System is hydrogen, with the remaining amount being mostly helium, oxygen and carbon. Everything else, like the metals and rocks is just a tiny fraction of a fraction of the mass in the Solar System.**
- **Since the Earth is constantly resurfacing itself, we can't find out how old it is, but there's another way to find out. Meteorites, which date back to the formation of the Solar System, have been raining down on Earth for millions of years. Scientists have sampled meteorites and learnt that they're all 4.6 billion years old. That means that everything in the Solar System formed are around the same time.**
- **Venus is the brightest planet in our sky and can sometimes be seen with the naked eye if you know where to look. It is the solar system's brightest planet – yellow clouds of sulphuric acid reflect the sun's light brightly.**

Chapter - 4

# THE SUN

The Sun is in the *centre of our Solar System* and is one of the *biggest stars in our galaxy*. It is made up of *hot gases that glow*. These gases are kept together on the sun's surface with the help of gravity. A major portion of these gases, nearly three-quarters, is **hydrogen**. The rest is mostly **helium** along with very small quantities of nearly 90 other elements.

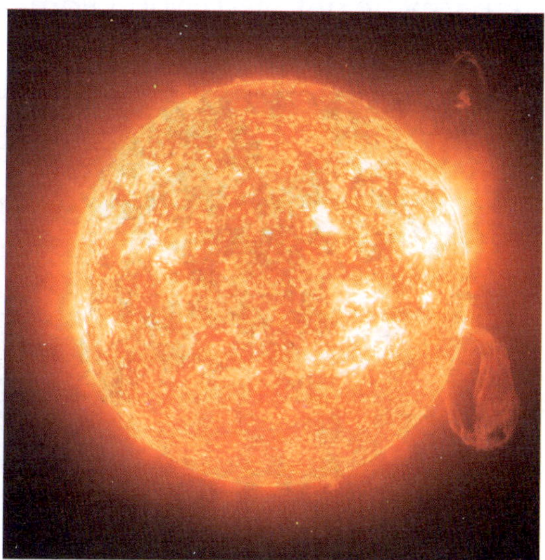

*Sun*

## Size

The sun is about *1.4 million kilometres (8,70, 000 miles) in diameter*. It is the largest body in the Solar System. While 1.3 million earths can fit inside the sun, 109 earths could fit across its face. It is made up of about 3,30, 000 times more material than that of the earth.

## Temperature

The sun is yellow in colour as its surface temperature is 5,500°C (9,900°F). While hotter stars are white in colour, the cooler ones are red. The core of the sun is 15 million°C (27 million°F). Here, 600 million tonnes of hydrogen is converted to helium every second with the help of nuclear reactions (the process of reacting various chemicals to produce nuclear energy).

## Spicules

Spicules are short-lived jets of gas which look like *flames*. These leap to a height of *10,000 kilometres (6,200 miles)* from the surface of the sun.

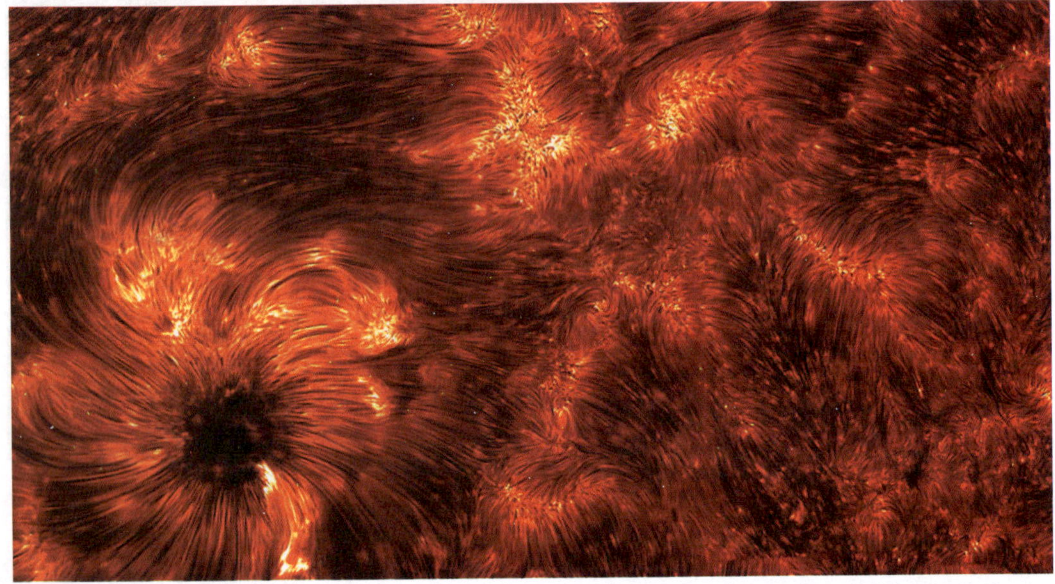

*Spicules*

## Atmosphere

The inner atmosphere of the sun, which lies directly above its surface, is known as the *chromosphere*. It extends to about *2,500 kilometres (1,550 miles)*. The chromosphere is followed by the *corona*. This extends to millions of kilometres into space.

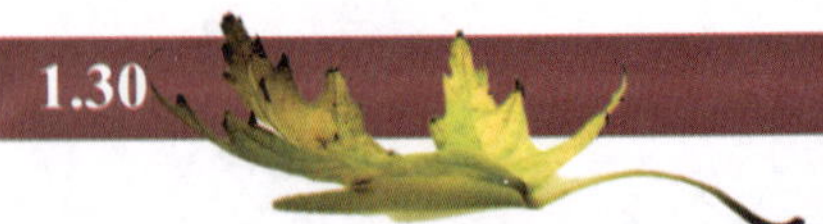

## Spin

As opposed to the spinning of the earth, different parts of the sun spin in different durations. While the regions near the poles take 30 days or more to complete one rotation, the equator completes it in 25 days.

### Quick Facts

- If the sun is seen from Mercury, it appears 2.5 times bigger than what it looks from the earth.
- Jupiter takes almost 12 years to orbit the sun.
- The sun is at a distance of 149 million kilometres from the earth.
- The sun comprises about 25% helium and 75% hydrogen.
- The sun is responsible for evaporation of about a trillion tons of water every day.
- A solar eclipse occurs when the moon is between the sun and the earth.
- The light from the sun reaches the earth in about eight minutes.
- The activity on the sun produces particles that are thrown out into space. This stream of particles, called the solar wind, consists primarily of protons and electrons and spreads throughout the solar system at about 450 km/sec. The solar wind has large effects on the tails of comets and the functioning of a spacecraft.
- Every second the sun loses 5 million tons of material and the sun's energy output is about 386 billion billion megawatts.

# Chapter - 5

# THE MOONS

All the planets in the Solar System, except Mercury and Venus, have their own satellites called the moons. There are more than 160 moons in the Solar System. All of these orbit around different planets.

The moons are of various sizes. Some are so huge that they are larger than Mercury, while some are only 2 kilometres (1.2 miles) across. Moons are generally made up of rock or rock and ice. Their surfaces have many impact craters (structures formed when a huge comet, asteroid or meteoroid crashes into a planet or a satellite). These were formed millions of years ago when the surface of the moons were hit by many asteroids (small solar bodies that orbit around the sun).

There are only nineteen moons in the Solar System that are more than 400 kilometres (250 miles) wide. While these moons are round in shape, smaller moons are irregular in shape.

## The Moon

The earth's moon is the fifth largest of all the

*Moon*

moons in the Solar System. It is the earth's only natural satellite and is about a quarter the size of the earth. Its surface does not have water and is covered with *impact craters*.

## IO

The most volcanic moon in the Solar System, *IO is very colourful*. Its surface is constantly renewed as molten rock erupts through its thin silicate-rock crust, and fast-moving columns of cold gas and frost grains shoot up from the surface cracks.

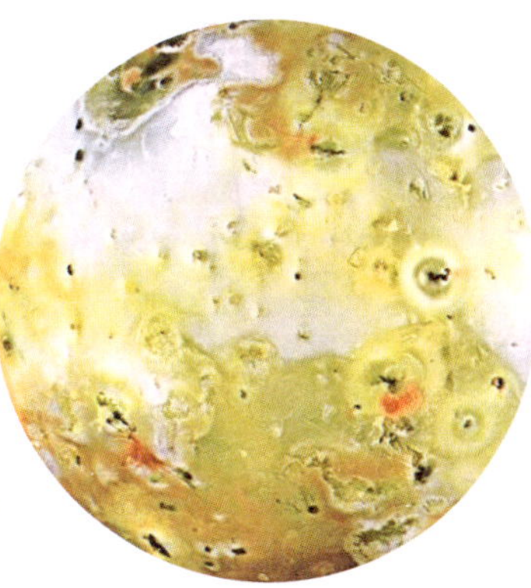

*IO*

## Europa

Europa is one of the four largest moons of Jupiter. The other three are *Io*, *Callisto* and *Ganymede*. Galileo Galilei was one of the first astronomers to see these four moons and so, together these four moons are called **Galileans**. Europa's surface has *brown grooves* that crisscross the blue-grey water ice.

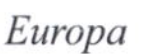

*Europa*

## Ganymede

Ganymede is the largest moon in the Solar System. It is one of Jupiter's moons and is about 5,262 kilometres (3,267 miles) in diameter. It is mainly made up of rock and ice, and has an *icy crust*. Till now, astronomers have found *63 moons around Jupiter*, but the number is increasing with astronomers finding more and more smaller moons.

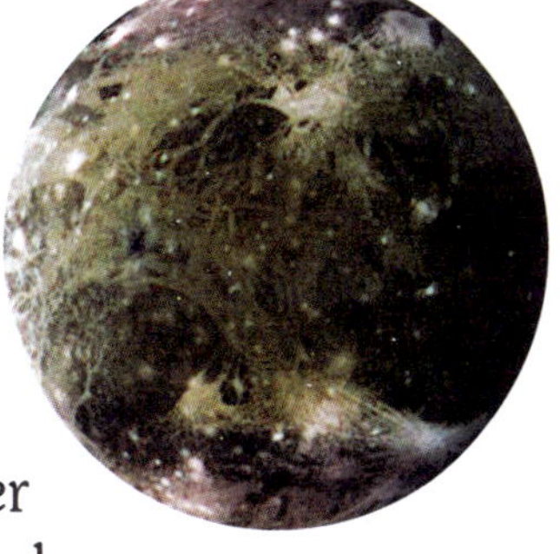

*Ganymede*

## Titan

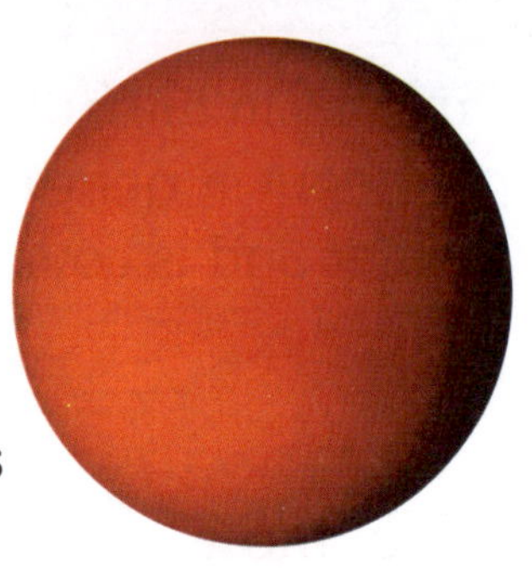
Titan

Saturn has *60 moons* and *Titan is the largest of them all*. Its surface is made up of seas, methane lakes, dark plains and bright highlands. It is the only moon which has an atmosphere, which is rich in nitrogen gas.

## Titania

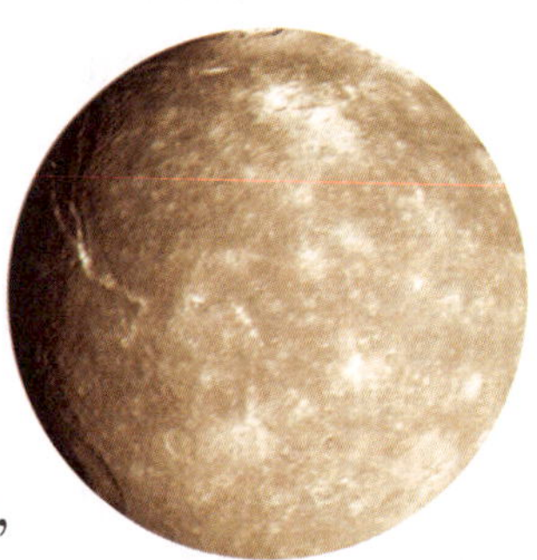
Titania

Uranus has *27 moons* and *Titania* is *the largest of them all*. Titania, along with other large moons of Uranus, such as Miranda, Ariel, Umbriel and Oberon, have got their names from characters in English literature. Titania has a grey, icy surface, with a lot of impact craters and large cracks.

## Triton

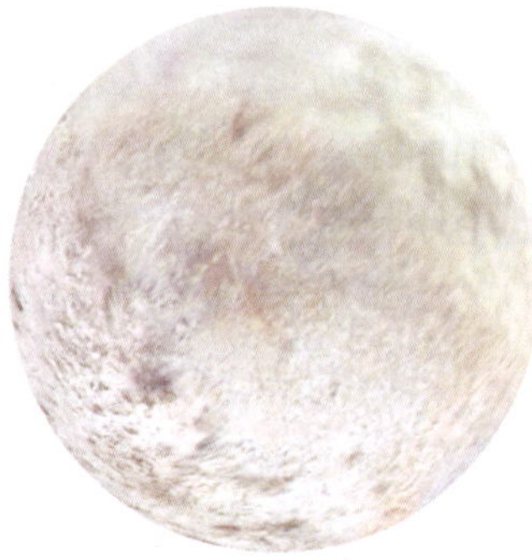
Triton

Out of Neptune's 13 moons, Triton is the largest. It is a ball made of rock and ice, with an icy surface. It is also called *cantaloupe* as its surface resembles a melon's skin.

## Small Moons

The Solar System has many small moons. Most of these are less than 400 kilometres (250 miles) across and irregular in shape. Quite a few of these have moons, such as the Mars has two moons, *Deimos* and *Phobos*, which started off as asteroids and later became moons.

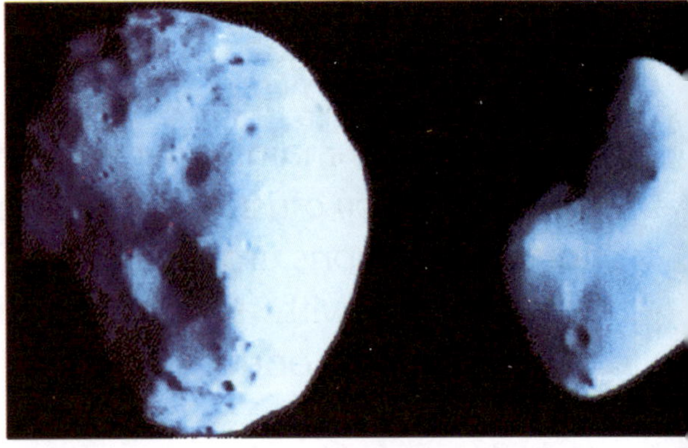
Small Moons

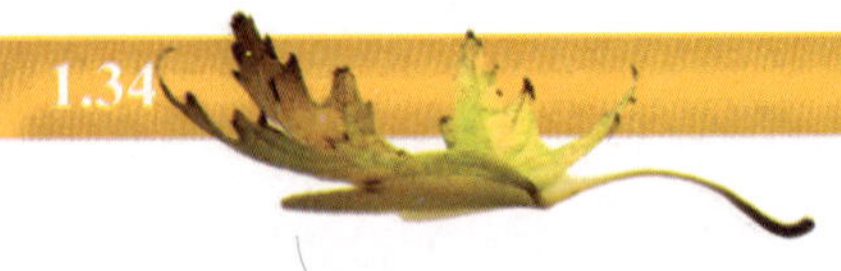

## Quick Facts

- It takes light about 1.5 seconds to reach the earth from the moon.
- The last man to land on the moon was Eugene Andrew Cernan in 1972.
- Neil Armstrong, the first person to walk on the moon, first put his left foot.
- A huge number of golf balls can be found on the moon as debris. Astronauts who have been to the moon and back used the balls for gravity experiments.
- The first person to walk on the moon was Neil Armstrong. The second was Edwin Aldrin.

# THE METEORITES

Millions of tonnes of rocky matter enter the earth's atmosphere every year. Most of it originates from asteroids, but some comes from other comets, the Moon, and even the Mars. When these rocky materials come close to the earth, they are called **meteoroids**. Generally, this rocky matter burns up, but if it does survive and land, it is called a **meteorite**.

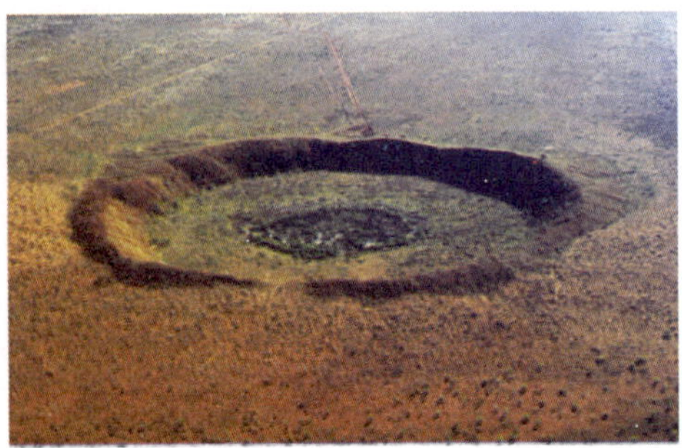

*Meteoroids*

Meteorites are generally of the following three types:

- Stony meteorites
- Iron meteorites
- Stony-iron meteorites (extremely rare)

## Meteor

Meteorites that burn in the atmosphere of the earth have *bright tails*. These short-lived streaks of light are termed as **meteors**, or **shooting stars**. About a million meteors occur every day.

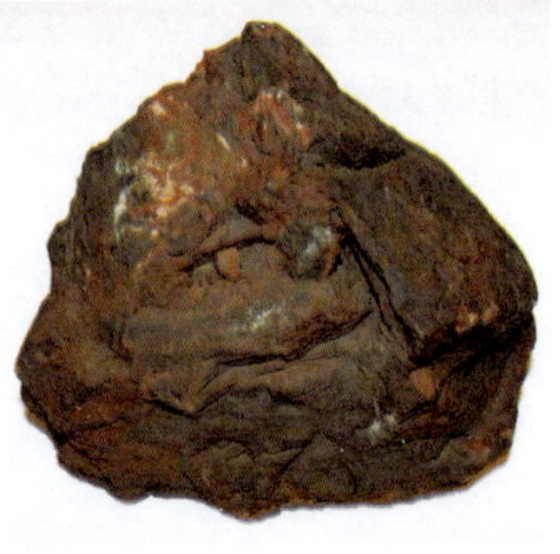

*Meteor*

## Esquel

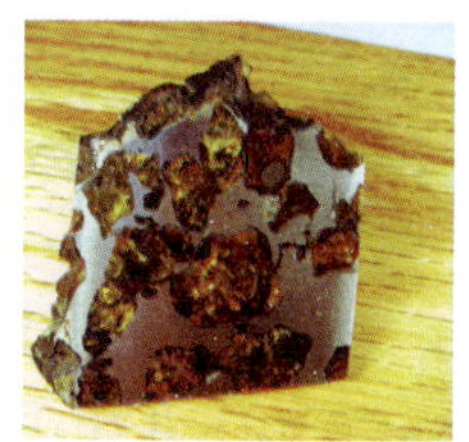

Esquel

Esquel is a rare stony-iron meteorite. It was found in 1951 in Esquel, Argentina. The iron-nickel metal of this meteorite has golden-coloured crystals of the olivine mineral embedded in it.

## Thiel

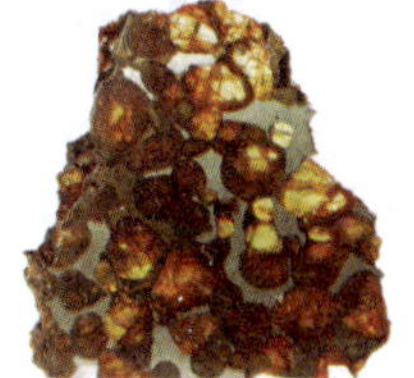

Thiel

Found in Antarctica, about 40 years ago, the Thiel Mountains have been formed by the stony-iron meteorites.

## Murchison

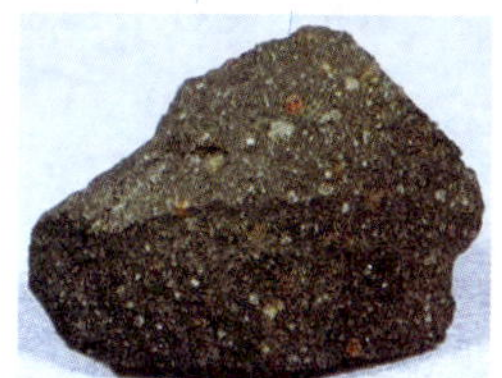

Murchison

Made up of water, minerals and various complex organic molecules, *Murchison is a stony meteorite*. It fell in *Australia in 1969* and has been thoroughly studied.

## Barwell

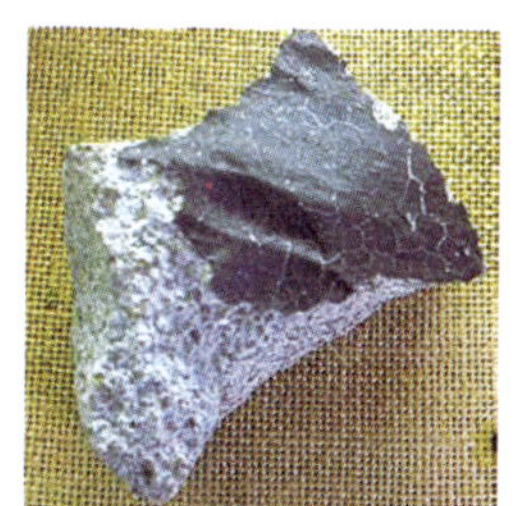

Barwell

In 1965, the *Barwell meteorite fell in England*. It was a part of a large shower of stones. When it entered the atmosphere of the earth, the friction caused the outer layer to heat up, and eventually, melt. After many years, it solidified and turned into a *black crust*.

## Canyon Diablo

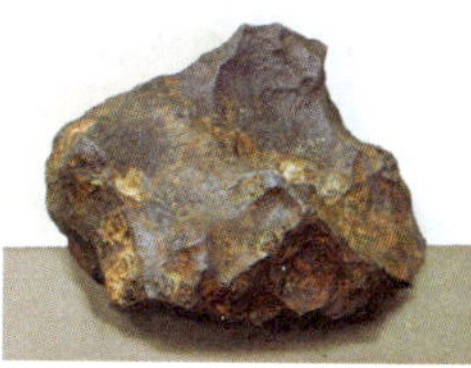

Canyon Diablo

Canyon Diablo is an *iron meteorite*. It is a sliced and polished piece of the asteroid which was responsible for producing the *Barringer Crater*. Even though the pieces found are only a tiny portion of the asteroid, together they weigh about 30 tonnes.

## Gibeon

After stony meteorites, iron meteorites are the second most commonly found. Gibeon is an *iron* meteorite. It is mainly made up of iron, but also has a small amount of *nickel* in it. It is one of the many *meteorites found in Namibia* since the 1830s.

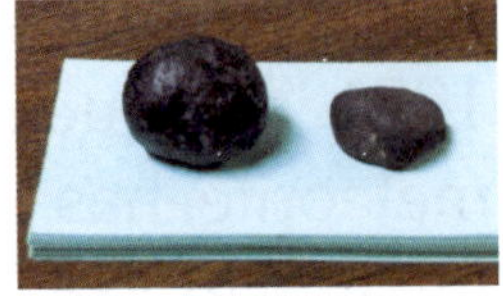

*Gibeon*

## Calcalong Creek

Quite a few of the meteorites found on the earth were formed when asteroids hit the moon. The *Calcalong Creek meteorite* is basically a *lunar surface soil* (soil that is found on the Moon) meteorite. It fell on the earth and turned into a rock due to the impact. It is located in *Australia*.

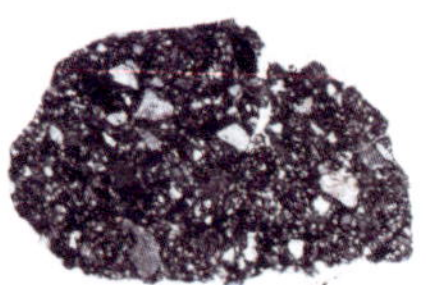

*Calcalong Creek*

## Nakhla

Nakhla is a *stony meteorite*. It is one of the many meteorites found on the earth, which originated on Mars. It landed in Egypt on 28th June 1911, before which it spent millions of years in the space after being blasted off from Mars.

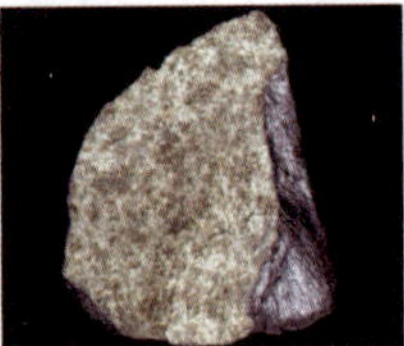

*Nakhla*

## Tektites

When a huge meteorite hits the earth, small glassy bodies can be formed. These are known as tektites. Due to the impact, the surrounding earth rock disintegrates and melts, and then is thrown upwards. When it cools down and becomes hard, it falls back on the earth as *glassy pieces*.

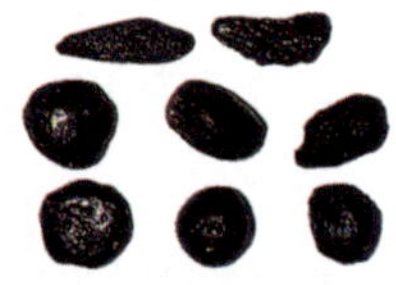

*Tektites*

## Impact Craters

Craters are formed when meteorites crash into the earth. These are usually very large in size. Formed about *50,000 years ago*, the

Barringer Crater in *Arizona Desert, USA*, measures 1.2 kilometres (0.75 miles) across.

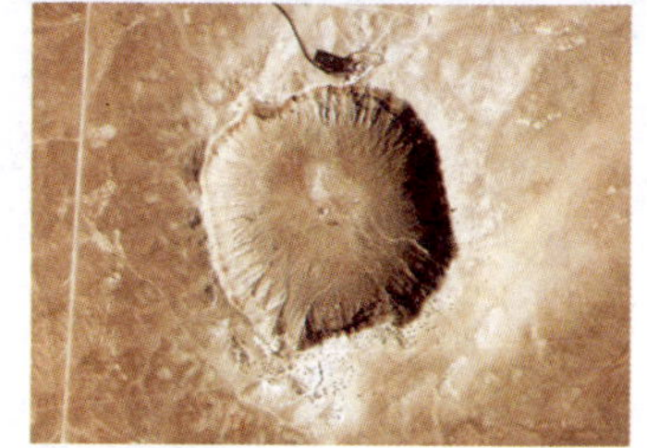

*Impact Craters*

## Quick Facts

- The asteroid belt is where the maximum meteorites come from.
- Meteorites fall under three major categories – Stone, iron and stone-iron.
- A meteorite is called a meteoroid before it enters the earth's atmosphere.
- The heaviest meteorite that fell on the earth weighed around 60 tonnes. It was called the Hoba West, and it fell in Africa.
- Meteor showers are periodic events. One can see thousands of meteors or shooting stars, as they are called, during such a shower. The most popular meteor showers are 'Perseids' (which peak around August 12) and 'Leonids' (which peak around November 17). During these showers, you can observe a shooting star at the rate of 1 meteor per minute on an average.
- Meteorites may look very much like earth rocks, or they may have a burnt appearance. They may be dense metallic chunks or more rocky. Some may have thumbprint-like depressions, roughened or smooth exteriors. They vary in size from micrometer size grains to large individual boulders.
- Some meteorites are sweet. They are made out of a substance similar to sugar.
- A falling meteor can travel at a speed of as much as 44 miles per second!
- Meteorites often contain minerals not found on the earth.

Chapter - 7

# THE COMETS

The planetary region in the Solar System is surrounded by more than a *trillion comets*. Like planets, *comets also orbit the sun*. All the comets together form a vast sphere known as the **Oort Cloud**.

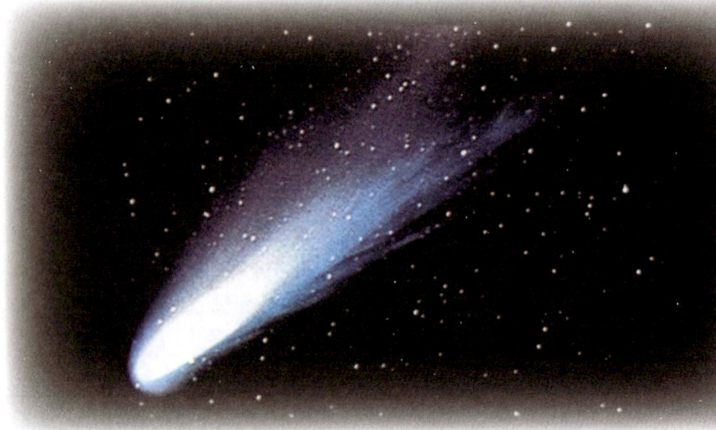

*Comets*

A comet is made up of a lump of *dirt and snow*. This lump is called a *nucleus* or dirty *snowball*. Very small in size, comets can be seen only when they travel very close to the sun as they become larger and brighter.

When a comet moves closer to the sun, it gets heated. All the snow in the comet starts turning into gas combined with the loose dust and begins to flow from the nucleus. When the comet passes closer to the sun than the orbit of Mars, this material forms a head (called a coma) and two tails, one of gas and one of dust.

Astronomers have identified more than **2,300 comets** that have passed through the sun's neighbourhood. While most of them just pass by, about 200 of these comets make return visits. Comets as magnificent as *Comet McNaught*, which was last seen in *January 2007*, can be seen only three to four times in a century.

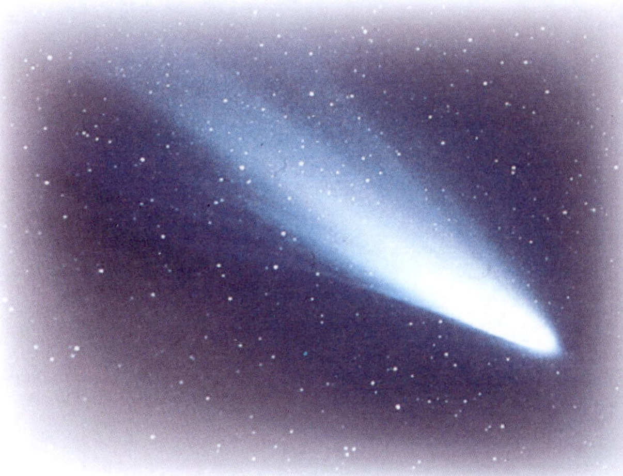

## Structure

The nucleus of a comet is made up of one-third rock dust and two-thirds snow.

## Breaking up

The gravitational force of huge bodies such as the Sun and Jupiter can pull a comet apart when it is passing them.

### Quick Facts

- **Comets are in orbit around the sun as are our planets.**
- **Comets are remnants from the cold, outer regions of the Solar System, which have been formed about 4.5 billion years ago.**
- **Comet orbits are elliptical. It brings them close to the sun and takes them far away.**
- **Short period comets orbit the sun every 20 years or less. Long period comets orbit the sun every 200 years or longer. Those comets with orbits in between are called Halley-type comets.**

- Comets have three parts: the nucleus, the coma and the tails. The nucleus is the solid centre component made of ice, gas and rocky debris. The coma is the gas and dust atmosphere around the nucleus. The tails are formed when energy from the sun turns the coma so that it flows around the nucleus and forms a tail behind it extending millions of miles through space.
- We see a comet's coma and tail because sunlight reflects off the dust (in the coma and dust tail) and because the energy from the sun excites some molecules so that they glow and form a bluish tail called an ion tail and a yellow one made of neutral sodium atoms.

# SPACE EXPLORATION

In the last five decades, humans have advanced technologically a great deal. They have been able to explore space with the help of spacecrafts. Within this short span of 50 years, more than 100 robotic crafts have been sent into space to explore various components of the Solar System. These include planets, stars, comets, asteroids.

## TIMELINE OF SPACE EXPLORATION

### October 14, 1957

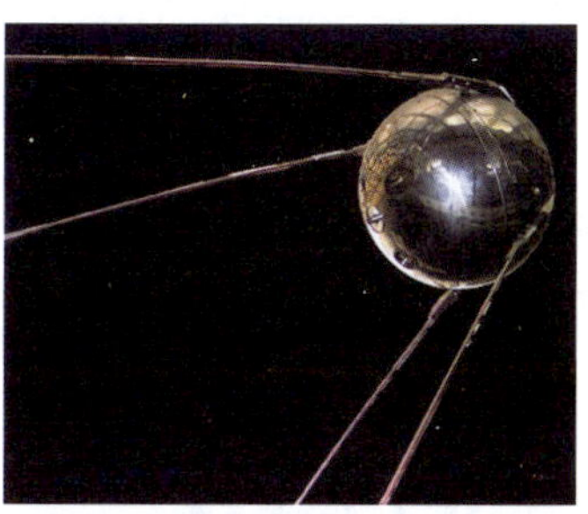

Russia launched the world's first artificial satellite, *Sputnik 1*, into the Earth's orbit.

### November 3, 1957

Sputnik 2 was launched into the Earth's orbit with a *Russian dog, Laika*, on board. This dog became the first creature to orbit the Earth.

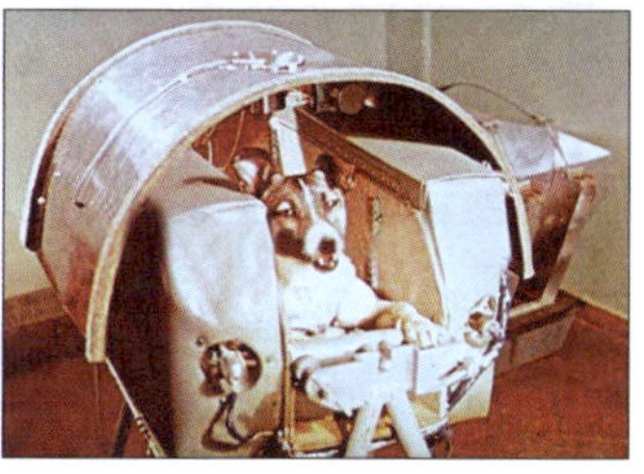

### January 2, 1959

*Luna 1, a Russian spacecraft*, became the first spacecraft to escape the Earth's gravity.

**September 13, 1959**

*Russian spacecraft, Luna 2*, was the first to land on the Moon. It crashed on its surface while landing.

**April 12, 1961**

*Yuri Gagarin*, a Russian cosmonaut, *became the first person to travel in space*. His flight lasted for about 108 minutes.

**June 16, 1963**

*Valentina Tereshkova*, a Russian cosmonaut, *became the first woman to go into the space.*

**March 18, 1965**

Another Russian astronaut, *Alexei Leonov*, became the first person to spacewalk (an astronaut's movement in the space outside the aircraft). Spacewalk is also known as Extra Vehicular Activity (EVA).

**February 3, 1966**

*Luna 9*, the space shuttle that successfully landed on the Moon.

**December 24, 1968**

US spacecraft *Apollo 8* became the first manned mission that left the Earth's gravity and orbited the Moon.

**July 20, 1969**

*Neil Armstrong and Buzz Aldrin* of Apollo 11 became the first human beings to walk on the Moon.

**April 19, 1971**

Russia launched the first space station – *Salyut 1*.

**December 3, 1973**

*Pioneer 10*, a US spacecraft, became the first craft to fly by Jupiter.

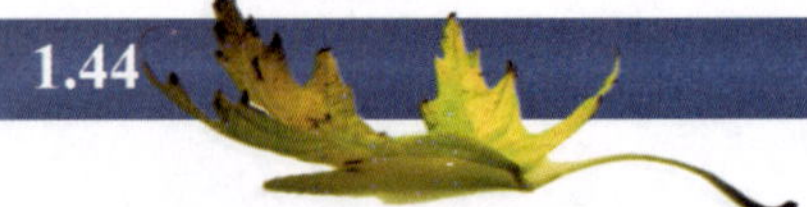

**March 29, 1974**

*Mariner 10*, another US spacecraft, became the first craft to fly by Mercury.

**July 17, 1975**

US craft *Apollo 18* and Russian *Soyuz 19* made the first international space rendezvous.

**October 22, 1975**

The first images from the surface of Venus were transmitted by the Russian spacecraft, *Venera 9*.

**July 20, 1976**

*Viking 1*, a US spacecraft, successfully landed on Mars.

**September 1, 1979**

US spacecraft *Pioneer 11* became the first to fly by Saturn.

**April 12, 1981**

Columbia, the first US space shuttle, was launched.

Launching of the first US space shuttle, Columbia

**January 24, 1986**

*Voyager 2*, a US craft, became the first to fly by Uranus.

**February 20, 1986**

The first module of Russian space station Mir was launched into orbit.

**March 13, 1986**

*Giotto*, a European spacecraft, became the first to take a close-up look at a comet.

**August 24, 1989**

The Hubble Space Telescope was launched.

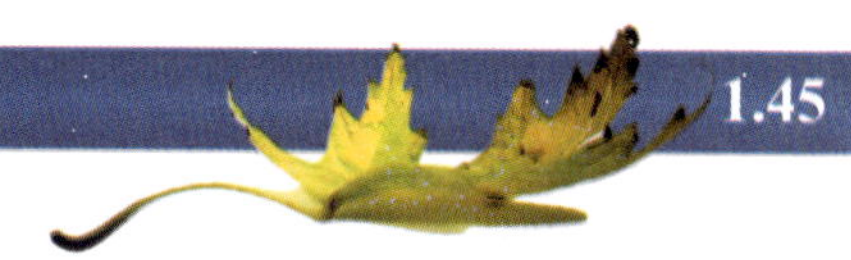

**September 15, 1990**

*Magellan*, a US spacecraft, began a three-year mapping programme of planet Venus.

**October 29, 1991**

*Galileo*, a US spacecraft, made the first flyby of an asteroid as it passed Gaspra.

**July13, 1995**

US spacecraft *Galileo* arrived at Jupiter. It then released a probe to enter Jupiter's atmosphere.

**July 4, 1997**

*Mars Pathfinder*, a US spacecraft, and its Sojourner rover landed on Mars.

**November 20, 1998**

The first module of the International Space Station (ISS), *Zarya*, was launched.

**February 12, 2001**

The Near Earth Asteroid Rendezvous (NEAR) Spacecraft landed on asteroid, *Eros*.

**August 25, 2003**

*Spitzer*, an infrared space telescope, was launched into the Earth's orbit.

**December 25, 2003**

Mars Express, Europe's first interplanetary craft, became the first to orbit Mars.

**January 4, 2004**

Mars Exploration Rover Spirit landed on Mars. It was followed by its twin, Opportunity.

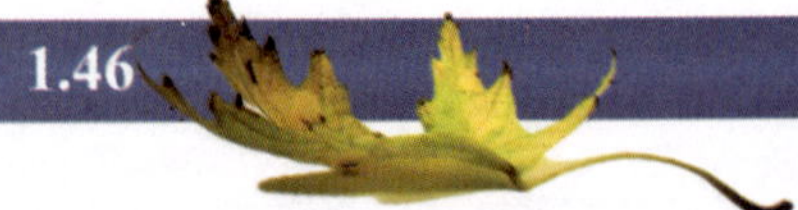

**March 2, 2004**

*Rosetta*, a European spacecraft, began its journey to Comet Churyumov-Gerasimenko. This journey would last for 10 years and carried lander Philae.

**June 30, 2004**

Cassini, a US craft, arrived at Saturn. The main aim of this journey was not only to study the planet, but also its moons. It released Huygens to land on the moon Titan.

**November 20, 2005**

*Hayabusa*, a Japanese spacecraft, landed on asteroid Itokawa.

**January 19, 2006**

New Horizons, a US craft, was launched on a journey to Pluto, which would last for eight years.

**August 4, 2007**

Phoenix, a US spacecraft, began its journey for Mars. It arrived there in 2008.

**January 14, 2008**

Messenger, a US spacecraft, made its *first flyby of Mercury*. This was a preparation before sending a craft to orbit the planet in 2011.

## Quick Facts

- There is no set number of people in an astronaut candidate class. The NASA selects its candidates on an as-needed basis. To even apply to be an astronaut, candidates must have completed 1,000 hours of flying time in a jet aircraft.
- A spacesuit weighs approximately 280 pounds—without the astronaut—and it takes about 45 minutes to put it on.
- Snoopy, from the Peanuts Comics, is the astronauts' personal safety mascot.
- Explorer 1, launched on January 31, 1958, was the first artificial satellite sent into space by the United States. It orbited the Earth every 115 minutes, and its cargo included a cosmic ray detector designed to measure the radiation environment in the Earth's orbit.

# PART - II

# THE EARTH

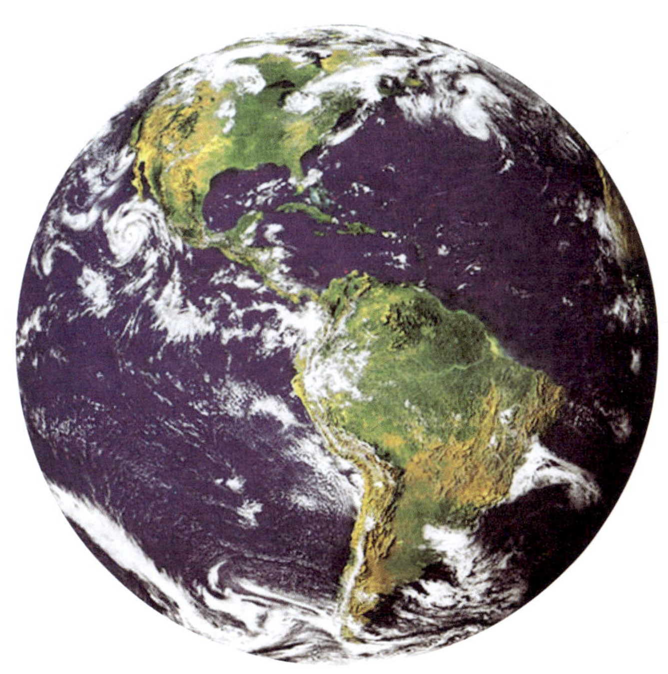

Chapter - 1

# THE PLANET, EARTH

The Earth was created about 4.5 billion years ago. It is made of a mass of rocky debris, rich in iron, which was orbiting the Sun. The rocks smashed into the young planet as meteorites, and were welded together by the heat generated from the energy of impact. This impact generated so much heat that the earth completely melted. Then the heavy iron sank towards the centre and became the core of the earth. The lighter rocks, on the other hand, became the **mantle** and the **crust**.

## Earth's Structure

The earth's structure resembles that of a *peach*.

- The centre of the earth is made up of *iron*. This metallic core resembles the hard stone which is at the centre of the peach.
- Then comes the hot, mobile rock of the mantle, which is just like the juicy flesh of the peach.
- Then at top is the earth's rocky crust, which is like the skin of the peach.

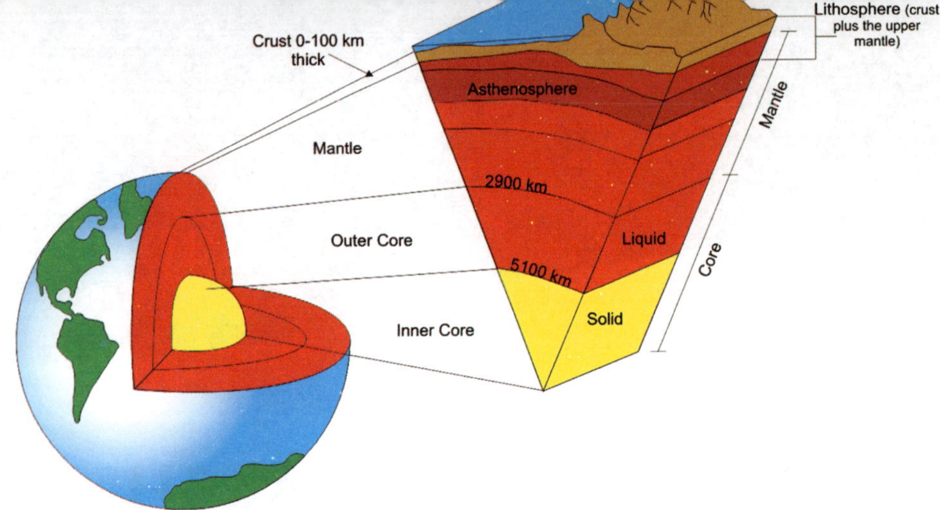


## Inner Core

The earth's inner core is a heavy ball made up of solid nickel and iron. Nuclear reactions within the earth heat it to about 4,700°C (8,500°F), but it does not melt due to the intense pressure at the core.

## Outer Core

A fluid mass of molten sulphur, nickel and iron surrounds the solid inner core of the earth.

## Lower Mantle

About 2,900 kilometres (1,800 miles) deep, the rocky mantle is heated to a temperature of about 3,500°C (6,300°F) at its base. Though it does not melt due to the intense pressure, the hot rock continues to move slowly due to the rising heat.

## Upper Mantle

The upper mantle is heated to almost 1,000°C (1,800°F). Wherever movement in the mantle causes the cool and brittle crust to crack, reduced pressure makes the hot mantle rock melt and erupt from the volcanoes.

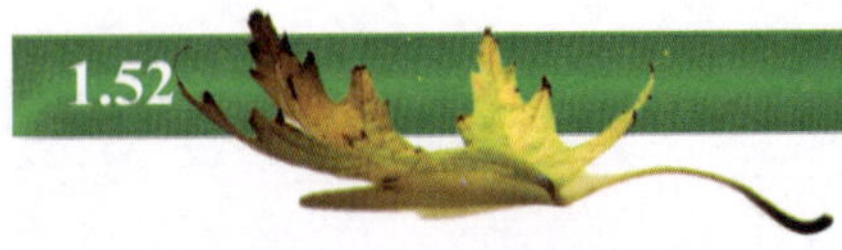

## Oceanic Crust

Oceanic crust, which lies between the continents, is less than 11 kilometres (7 miles) thick. Made of heavy rocks that erupt from the hot mantle at mid-ocean ridges, it forms the bedrock of the ocean floors.

## Continental Crust

The lightest rocks of the earth combine and form *large slabs*. They float on the mantle, which is quite heavy. Nearly 70 kilometres (45 miles) thick, they rise above the sea level and form the continents we live on.

## Land Surface

*Sunlight, rain, wind and frost* breakdown the rocks on land. This exposure to erosion (process of removal of the earth's top layer) and weathering (*breakdown* of rocks, minerals and soils as a result of contact with the earth's atmosphere) releases minerals which are essential for the survival of various plants and other life forms.

## Oceans

The areas lying between the continents are filled with *large masses of water called the oceans*. Most of the water erupted from volcanoes as water vapour early in the earth's history. They caused torrential rains which resulted in the formation of rivers, seas and oceans. Even the melting of ice resulted in the formation of oceans.

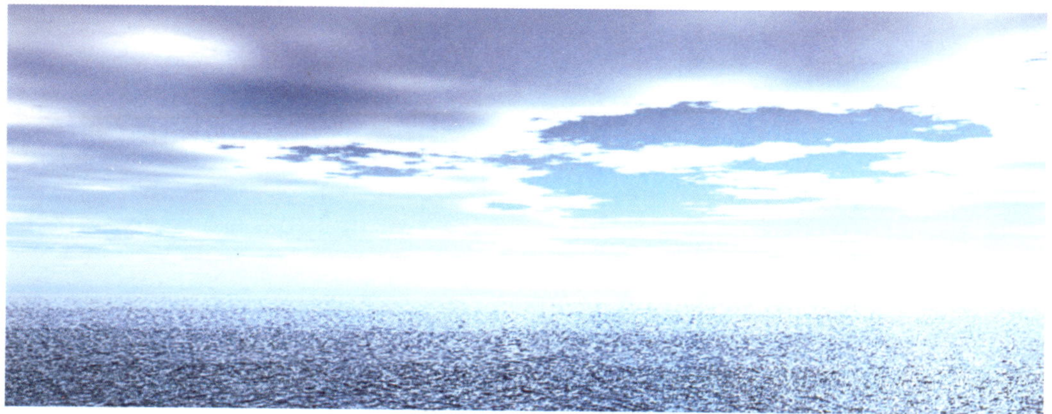

## Weather Systems

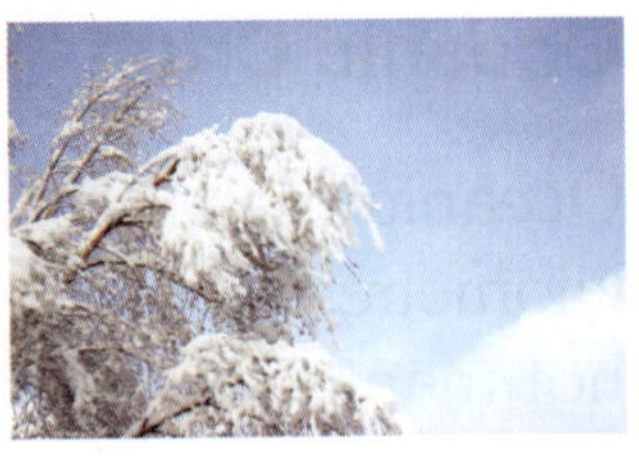

Due to the sun's heat, the water vapour from the oceans rise into the lower atmosphere. This water gets collected and forms large masses of clouds. The clouds then spill rain onto the continents, allowing life to exist on land.

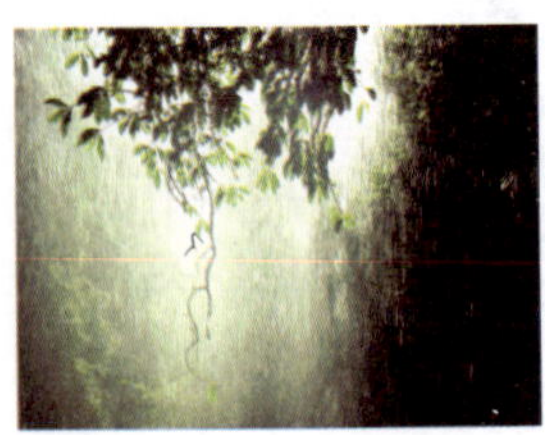

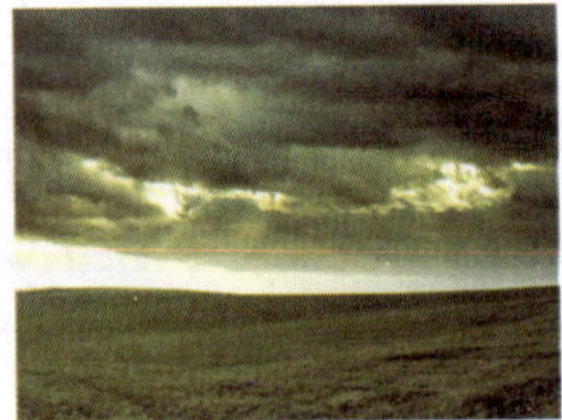

## Atmosphere

The earth's atmosphere is made up of many gases including *oxygen*, *carbon dioxide* and *nitrogen*. This atmosphere not only keeps the earth warm at night, but also protects it from dangerous radiations.

## On the Surface

The earth's thin and cool crust has been broken up into many huge plates due to the movements in the hot and thick mantle. The boundaries of these plates are marked by earthquake zones dotted with volcanoes, and mountain ridges pushed up, where moving plates collide.

### Quick Facts

- **The crust of the Earth is a very small part of its vast mass.**
- **The heat that rises from the mantle pushes the plates of the crust apart.**
- **Mountains are formed whenever the oceanic crust is dragged beneath the continents.**
- **More than 70 percent of the earth's surface is made up of ocean water.**

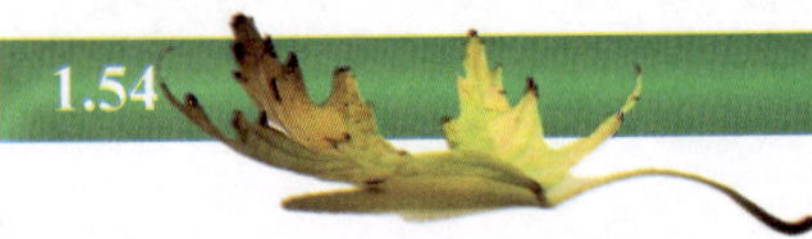

Chapter - 2

# PLATE TECTONICS

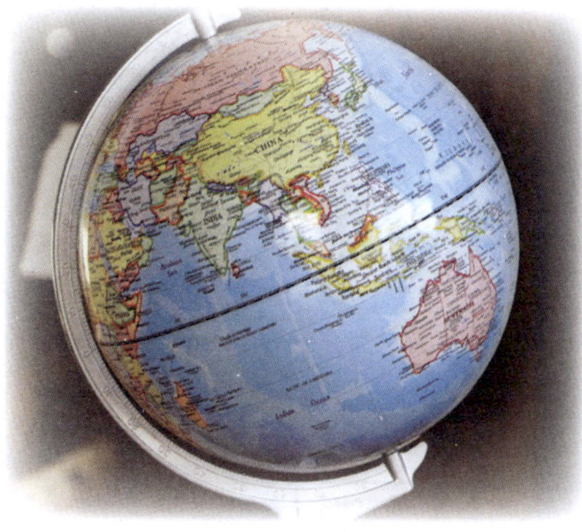

The outer covering of the earth is a *brittle shell*, known as the **crust**. Below the crust is a deep layer of hot rock called the **mantle**. The heat produced within the earth makes the mantle move, but very slowly. This movement makes the crust crack and break up into separate plates, which are being pushed together in some places and pulled together in others. When the plates move, they carry the continents around the globe, and also make oceans smaller or larger.

## Parts

There are about *40 small tectonic plates* and *15 large ones*. They form the ocean floors, and some of the largest even carry the *continents*. The rocks from which continental plates are made are thicker, but much lighter, than the rocks of the ocean floor. The continents continue to move, but unlike the oceanic parts of the plates, they do not usually change the shape and size.

## Plate Boundaries

The plate boundaries are at some places pushed together, while at others, they are pulled apart. It might even be possible sometimes that one plate slides against another. Many plate boundaries are dotted with volcanoes, which may go off due to such movement. Earthquakes are also a result of these movements.

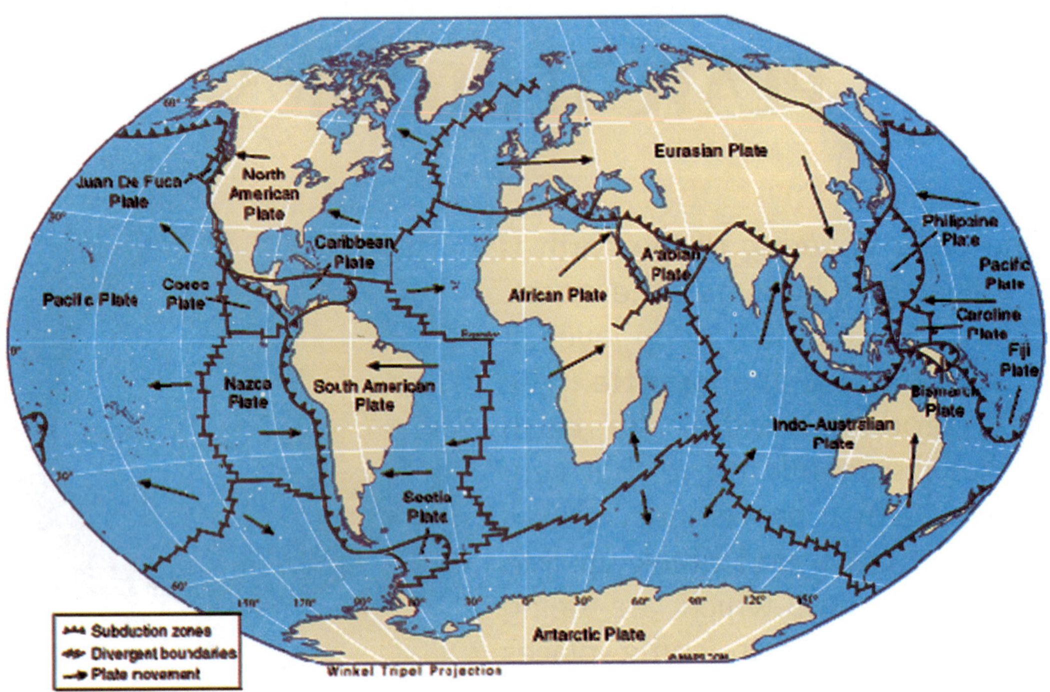


## Convergent Boundaries

Convergent boundaries are found where a plate slides under another. For instance, ocean floors grind under continents. Due to this, mountain ranges are pushed up.

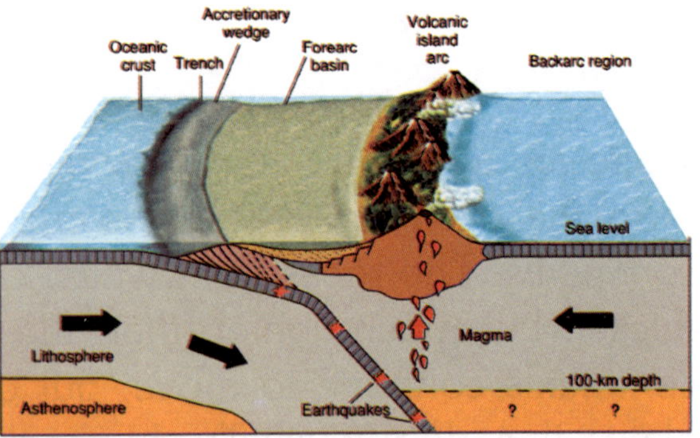

## Divergent Boundaries

Divergent boundaries are formed where the plates pull apart. This usually occurs on the ocean floors. As the plates are pulled apart, the hot mantle rock erupts in the rift zone and then solidifies as the new **ocean floor**.

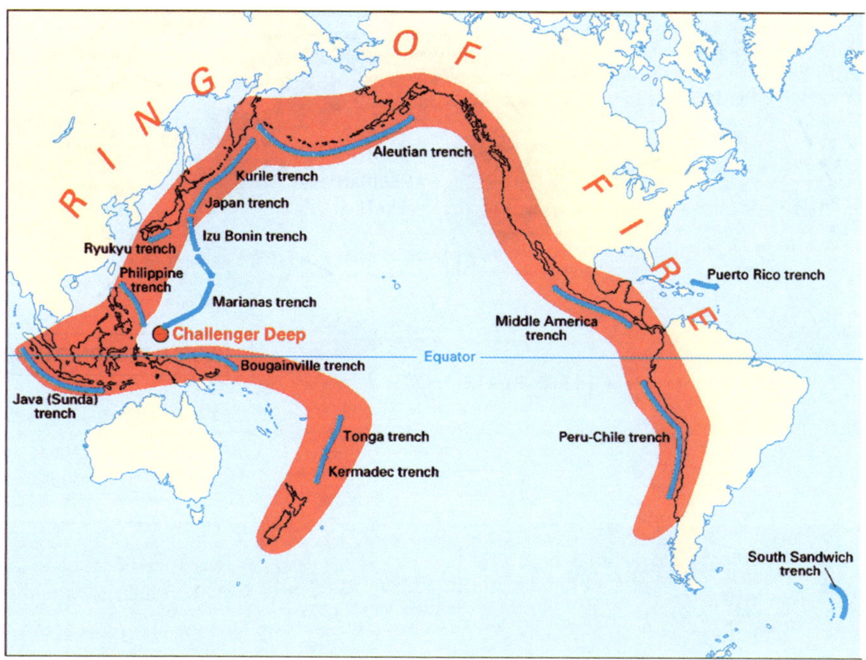


## Transform Boundaries

Transform boundaries are formed where two plates slide past each other. This causes frequent **earthquakes** along the *fault line* (a crack in the earth's surface usually caused by earthquakes).

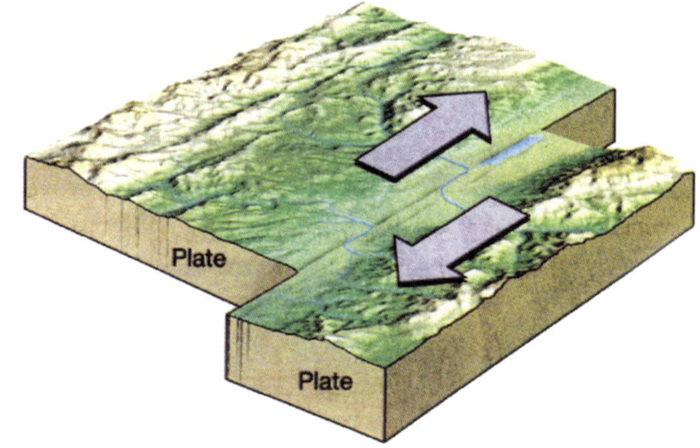

## Globe

All the plates fit together perfectly to form the globe.

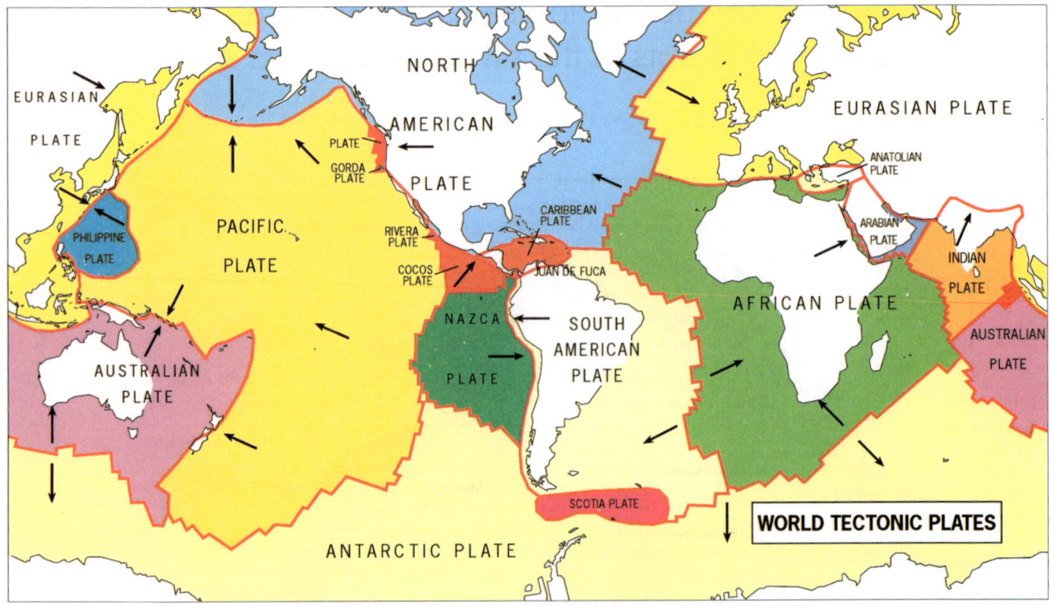


## Quick Facts

- Convergent tectonic plates move towards one another and the Divergent plates separate from each other.
- Transform plates slide together in a horizontal, vertical, or diagonal way.
- Every year, the seven continents move approximately 2 centimetres away from each other.
- Earthquakes are caused from transform plates.
- Some parts of the earth are either splitting or coming near each other.

# EARTHQUAKES

The large plates of the earth's crust move continuously. Earthquakes take place when these plates meet and cause movement. Minor movement, that may even occur frequently, just causes **tremors** or shaking of the Earth, but what generally happens is that the rocks on the boundaries of each plate get locked together. The strain keeps on building up till the rocks get distorted and the locked section gives way. The rock then springs back, often shifting several metres, and the shock of this can cause a **disastrous earthquake**.

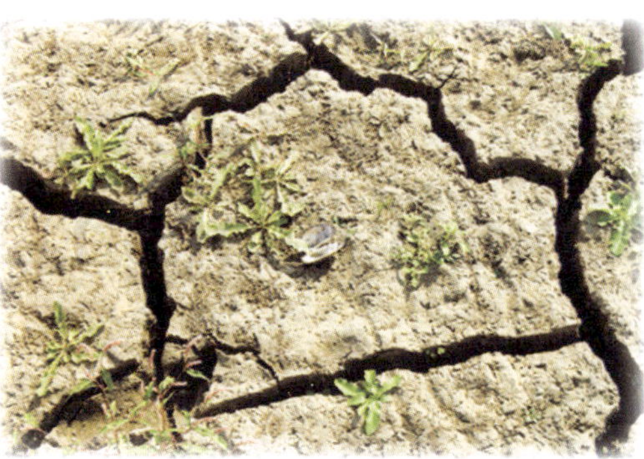

*Earthquakes*

Earthquakes are recorded with the help of an instrument called the **seismograph**. It was devised by the **American scientist, Charles Richter in 1935**.

## Chile, 1960

The biggest earthquake to be recorded in history struck **Chile** in **1960**. It reached *9.5 on the Richter Scale*.

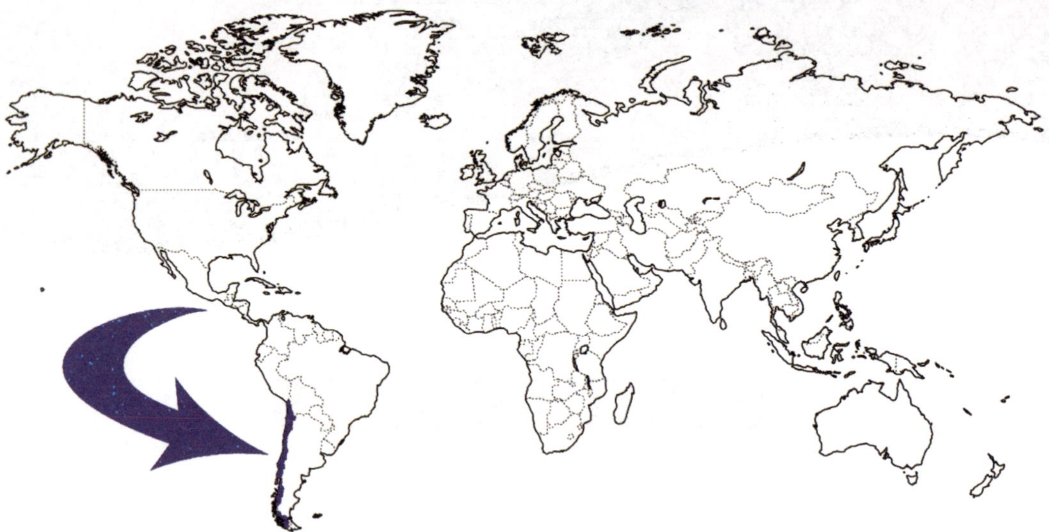

## Alaska, 1964

In this huge earthquake, within a span of a few minutes, the Pacific Ocean floor slid 20 metres (66 feet) beneath Alaska. Not too many lives were lost as very few people stay in this region.

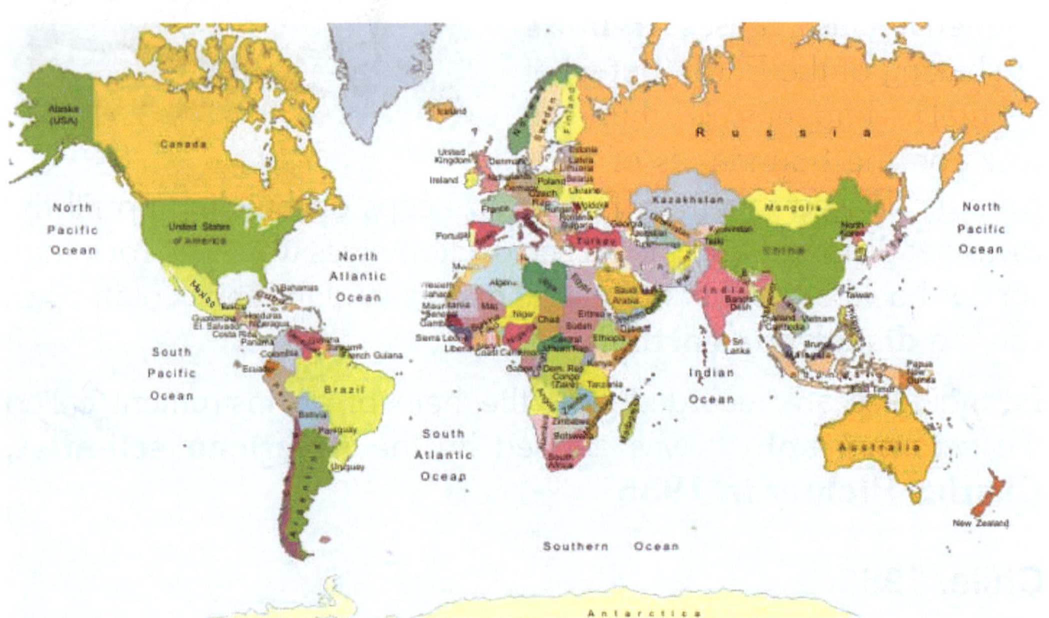


## Mexico City, 1985

In 1985, a massive earthquake shook the city of Mexico. Over 400 multi-storeyed buildings were destroyed, and the death toll crossed 9,000.

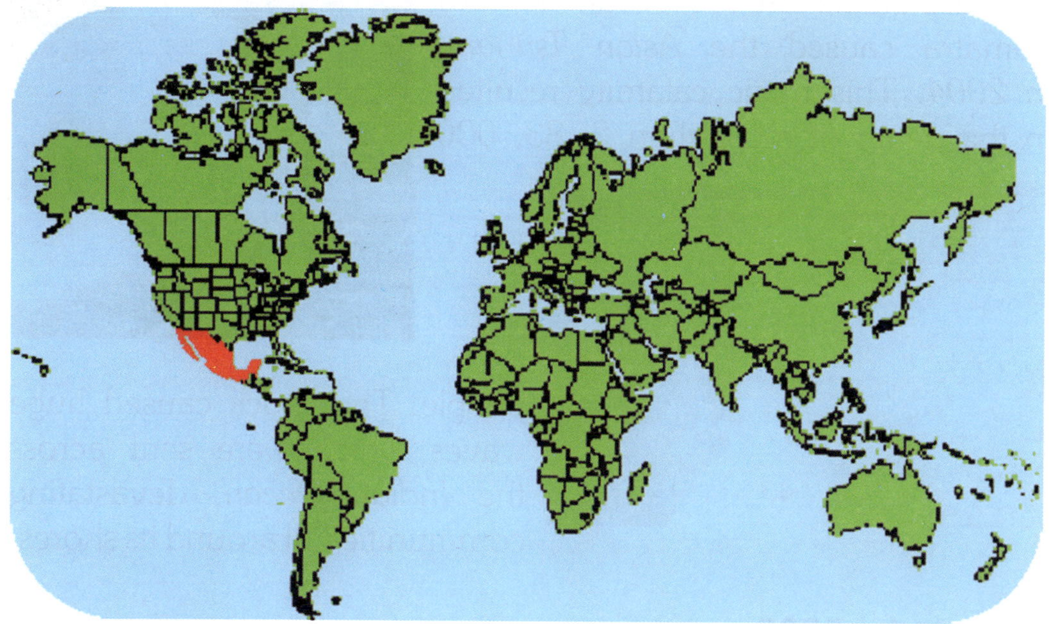

## Kobe, 1995

*Japan has more earthquakes* than any other place on the earth. *Kobe, a city in Japan*, was severely damaged by a serious earthquake in 1995. It also resulted in the death of about 6,433 people.

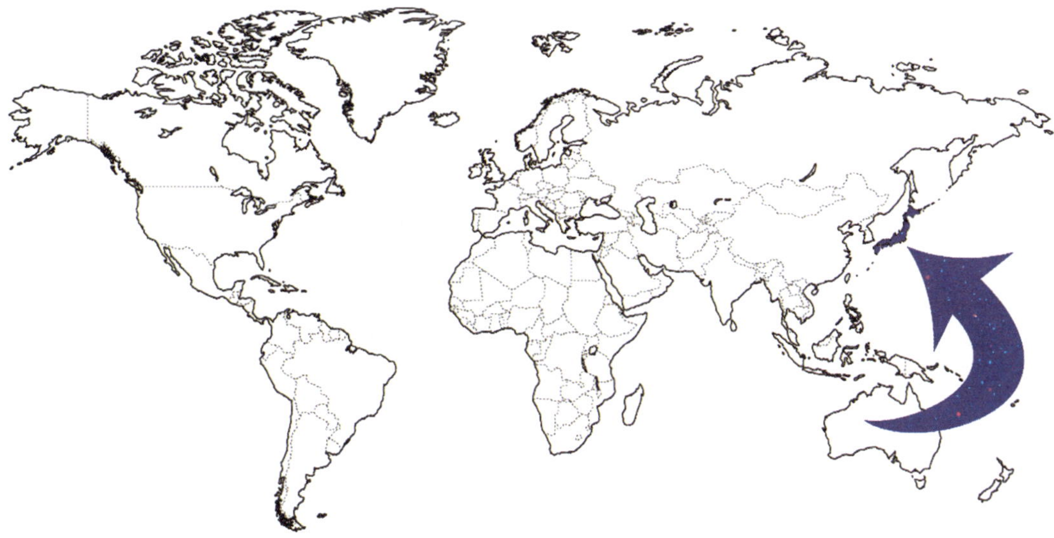

## Tsunami, 2004

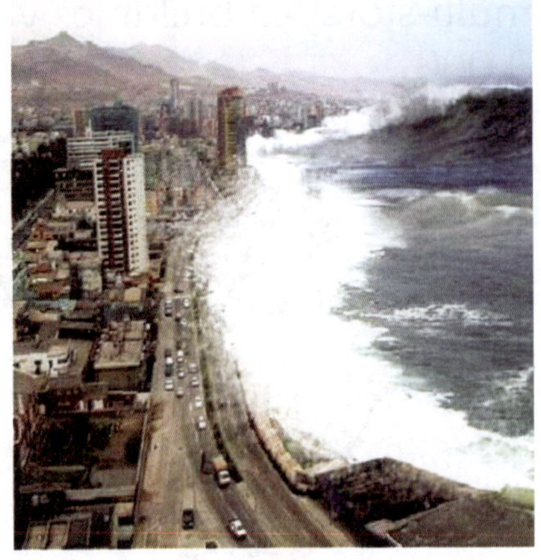

An earthquake on the ocean floor of Sumatra caused the *Asian Tsunami in 2004*. This tragic calamity resulted in the death of more than 2, 83, 000 people. The shock caused huge waves which were sent across the *Indian Ocean*, devastating communities all around its shores.

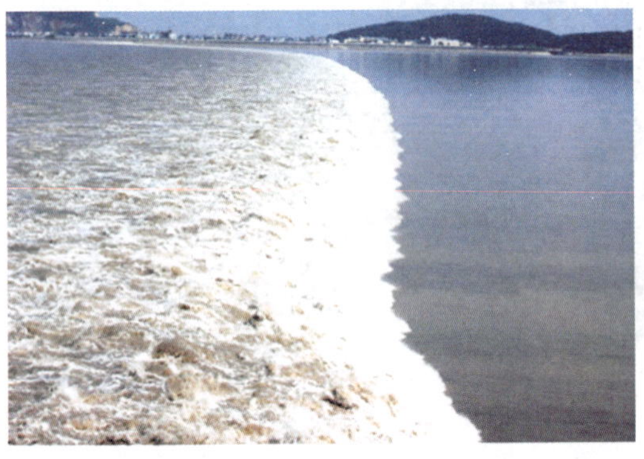

## Indonesia, 2006

A disastrous earthquake hit the island of **Java** in **2006**. It not only destroyed 1, 35, 000 houses, but also killed at least 5,780 people. A World Heritage site, the ancient **Hindu temple of Prambanan**, was also damaged but wasn't destroyed.

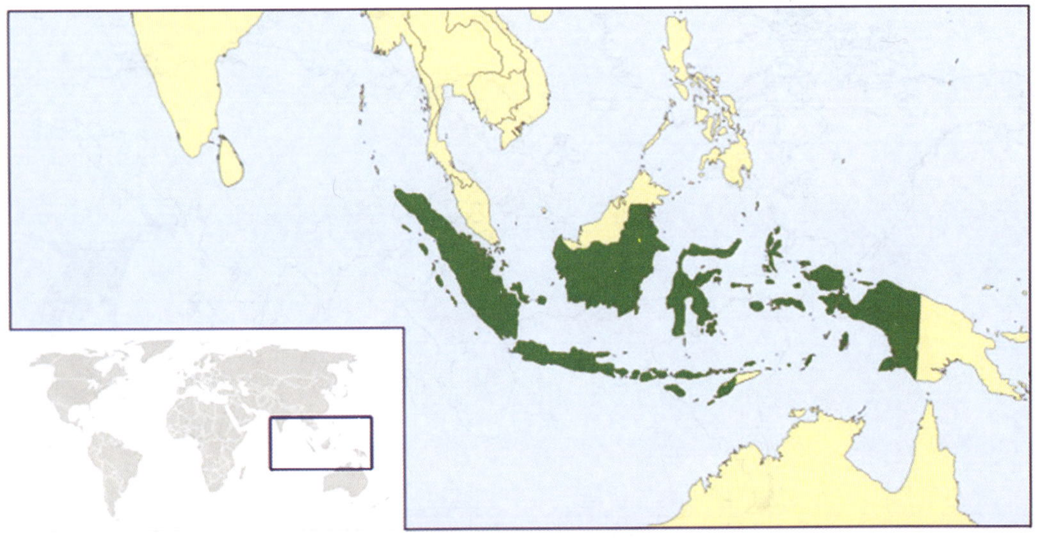

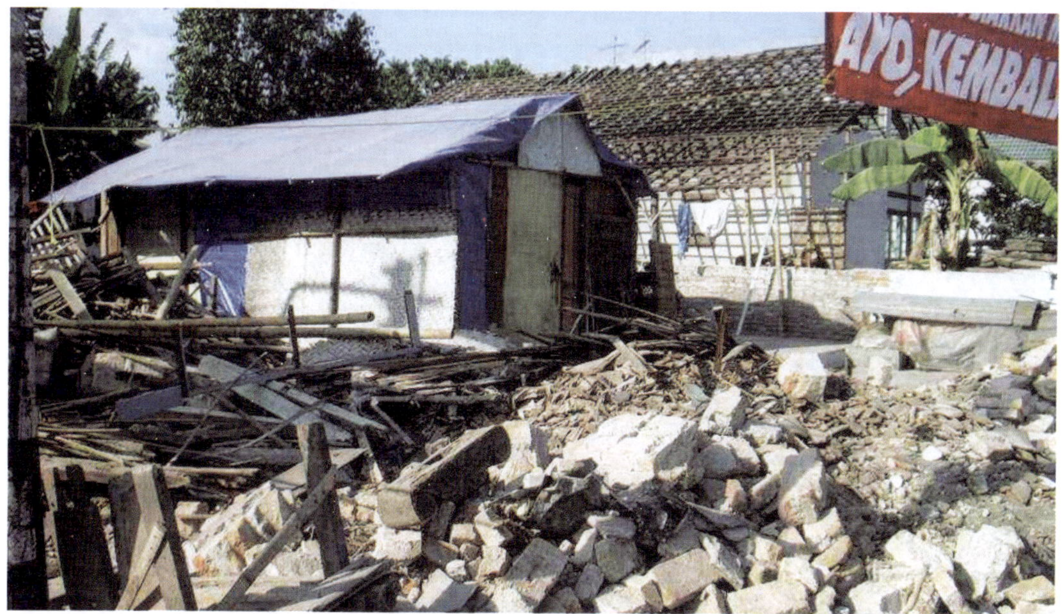


*The Aftermath of the Earthquake in Indonesia, 2006*

## Quick Facts

- Earthquakes cause vibrations, and a seismograph machine records the motion of the ground during a quake. Scientists cannot predict a quake, but they can detect smaller regional vibrations along known as fault lines that may indicate that a bigger quake is coming.
- Since 1900, the largest measured earthquake on record was a magnitude of 9.5 in the Richter Scale in Chile on May 22, 1960. The second-largest was a magnitude of 9.2 in the Richter Scale in Alaska on March 28, 1964, the biggest ever in the United States.
- A Tsunami is a sea wave caused by an underwater earthquake or landslide and a tidal wave is a large sea wave produced by high winds.

- It is estimated that there are about 500,000 detectable earthquakes in the world each year. About 100,000 can be felt by humans, and around 100 of them cause various degrees of damage.
- Sometimes, there are many small earthquakes before the big one. These small ones are called foreshocks. However, sometimes, after the big earthquake, the main shock, again there may be many small quakes. These are called the aftershocks.
- Many earthquakes happen on the ocean floor. Big ocean waves can form after a quake resulting in a Tsunami.
- The shaking of the ground is not what kills most victims of earthquakes. The main killers in earthquakes are falling buildings, fires, landslides, avalanches and Tsunamis.
- An earthquake happens somewhere in the world once every thirty seconds.
- You may not notice a magnitude 2 quake. You would feel the ground shake in a magnitude 3 quake. A magnitude 7 or higher can destroy a city.

# Chapter - 4

# THE VOLCANOES

The word, *volcano* is derived from the name of Vulcano, a *volcanic island in the Aeolian Islands of Italy* whose name in turn originates from Vulcan, the name of a *God of fire in Roman mythology*.

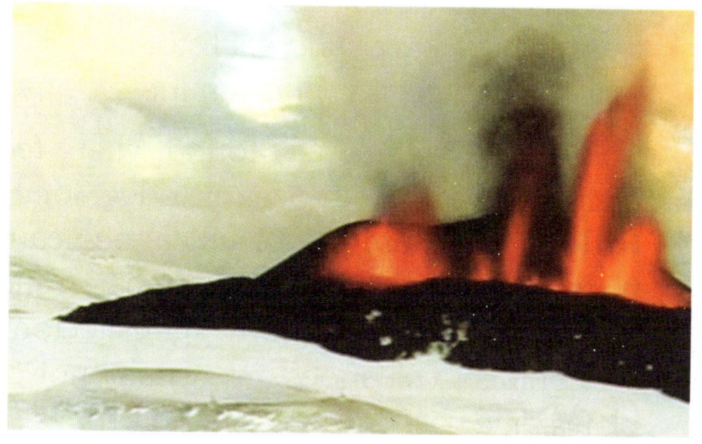

*Volcano*

Volcanoes are the most destructive of all the geological features of the earth. Generally, volcanoes are located along the boundaries of the plates, where the rocks that make up the crust of the earth meet. Friction of plates grinding against each other and opening rifts make the hot rock beneath the crust melt and burst up through **fissures** (cracks). Volcanoes may also occur over hotspots away from the plate boundaries, caused by the rising plumes of heat in the mantle beneath the earth's crust.

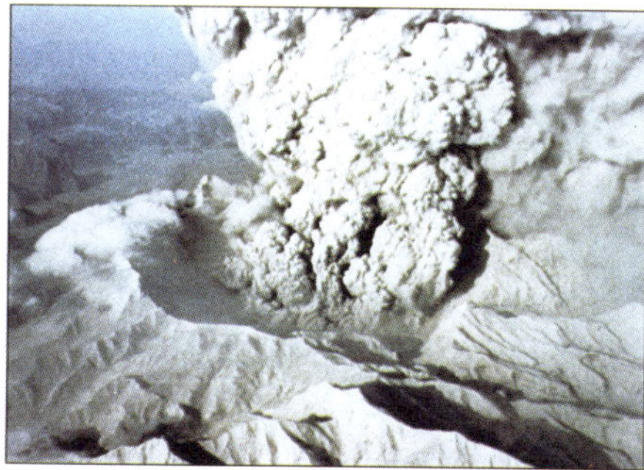

*Fissures*

A volcano is basically an opening, or rupture, in a planet's surface or crust, which allows hot **magma**, **volcanic ash** and **gases** to escape from below the surface.

Ash **plumes** reached a height of about 19 km during a *volcanic eruption at Mount Pinatubo, Philippines in 1991*.

Erupting volcanoes can pose many hazards, mainly in the immediate vicinity of the eruption. Volcanic ash can be a threat to aircraft, particularly those with jet engines where ash particles can be melted by the high operating temperature. Large eruptions can affect temperature as ash and droplets of sulphuric acid obscure the sun and cool the **earth's lower atmosphere or troposphere**. However, they also absorb heat radiated up from the earth, thereby warming the *stratosphere*. Historically, the so-called *volcanic winters* have caused *catastrophic famines*.

Volcanoes are generally found where *tectonic plates are diverging or converging*. A mid-oceanic ridge, for example, the **Mid-Atlantic Ridge**, has examples of volcanoes caused by divergent tectonic plates pulling apart and the Pacific Ring of Fire has examples of volcanoes caused by convergent tectonic plates coming together. By contrast, volcanoes are usually not created where two tectonic plates slide past one another. Volcanoes can also form where there is stretching and thinning of the earth's crust in the interiors of plates, e.g., in the East African Rift, the Wells Gray-Clearwater Volcanic Field and the Rio Cleveland Volcano in the Aleutian Islands of Alaska and the Grande Rift in North America. This type of volcanism falls under the umbrella of "Plate hypothesis" volcanism. Volcanism away from plate boundaries has also been explained as **mantle plumes**. These so-called 'hotspots', for example, Hawaii, are postulated

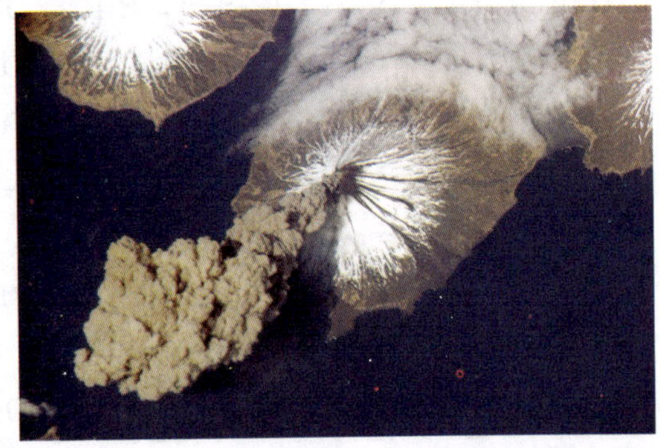

to arise from upwelling diapirs with magma from the core-mantle boundary, 3,000 km deep in the earth.

The study of volcanoes is called **Volcanology**, sometimes spelled **Vulcanology**.

## Quick Facts

- The gas clouds that are a result of volcanic eruptions are mainly made of sulphur dioxide, water vapour and carbon dioxide.
- Lava bombs are cooled down forms of the molten rocks that erupt from volcanoes.
- Lava flows downhill at the speed of up to 100 kilometres per hour (60 miles per hour).
- The lava that erupts glows and is bright orange in colour because of its immensely high temperature of approximately 1,000°C (1,830°F).
- A hundred kilometres an hour is the approximate speed of the molten lava that flows downhill.



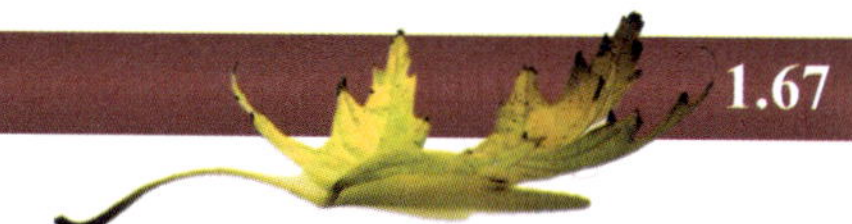

Chapter - 5

# THE MOUNTAINS

When the plates of the earth's crust grind together, the edges of the continental plates are pushed up into *high, folded ridges*, called the *mountains*. When hot rock from beneath the surface erupts through the cracks in these mountains, *volcanoes* are formed.

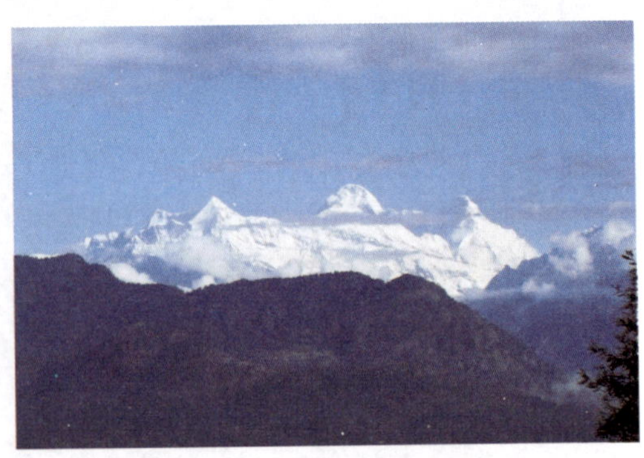

## Mount Everest

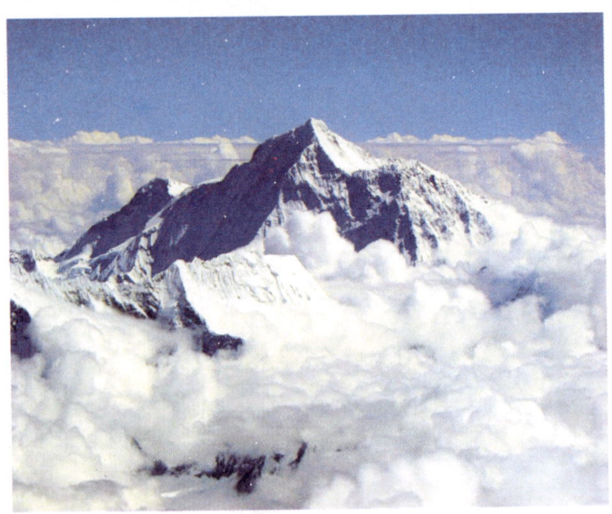

Lying around *8,850 metres (29,035 feet) above the sea level*, *Mount Everest* is the highest peak in the world. It is a part of the *Himalayan range*, which lies in India. These mountains were formed *50 million years ago*, when India collided with Asia.

## Mount Aconcagua

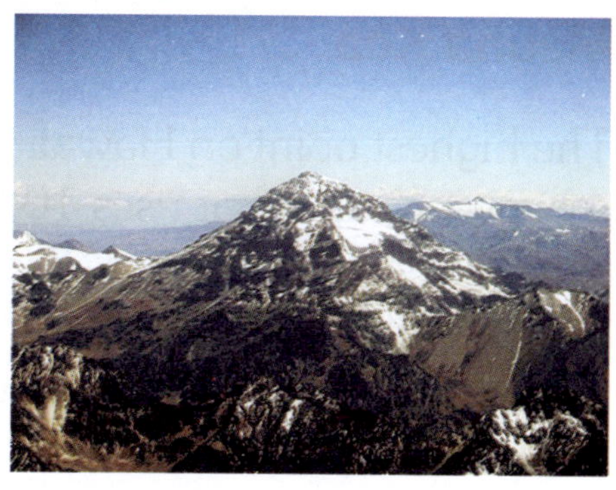

Mount Aconcagua is the highest peak of the Andes mountain range,

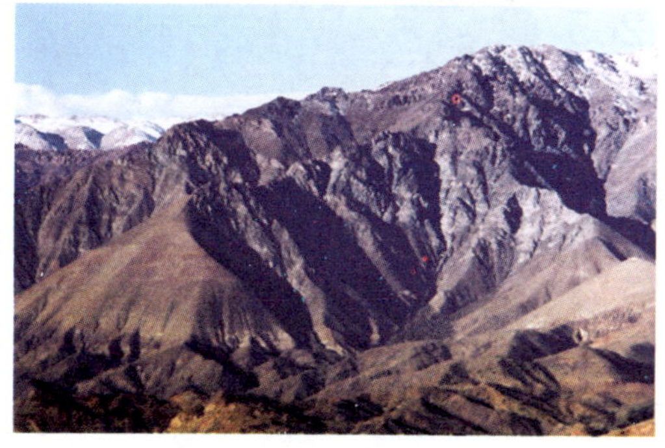

which lies in South America. Its height is about 6,959 metres (22,834 feet). This mountain range is very prone to earthquakes.

## Mount McKinley

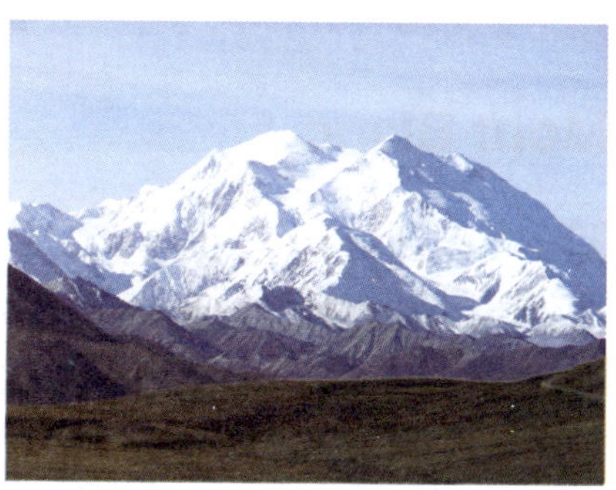

The highest peak of North American Western Cordillera, Mount McKinley, is around 6,194 metres (20, 321 feet) above the sea level. It is located in Alaska, and due to its isolation it is one of the most remarkable mountains of the world.

## Mount Kilimanjaro

*Mount Kilimanjaro is the highest peak in Africa.* In reality, it is not a mountain, but a *huge volcano* with three volcanic cones. Out of the peaks of the three cones, the tallest is **Kibo**, which rises about 5,895 metres (19,340 feet) above the sea level. The other two cones are called *Shira and Mawenzi*.

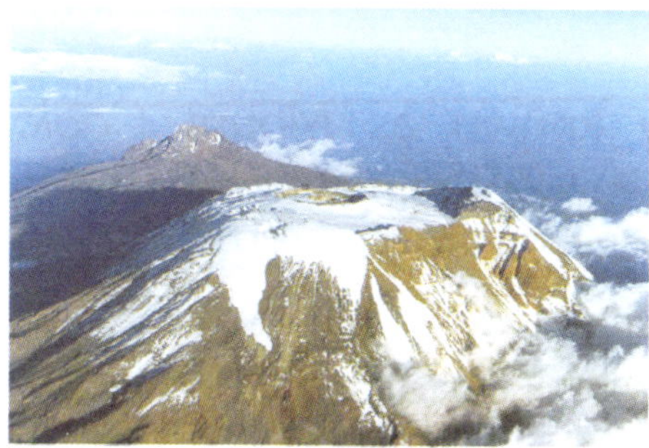

## Mauna Kea

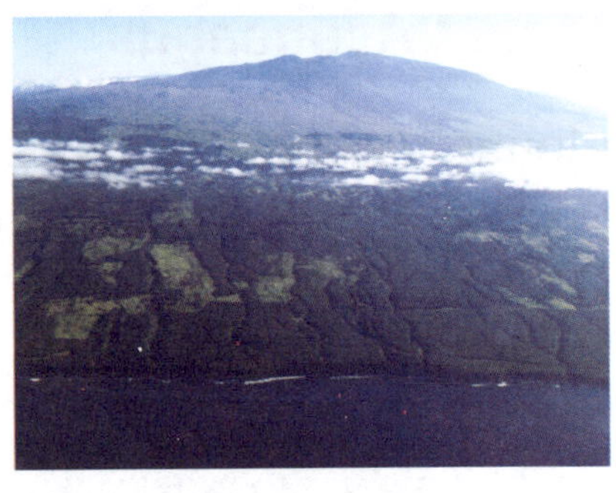

The highest point on Hawaii is the top of a huge volcano that rises 10,000 metres (33,000 feet) from the Pacific Ocean floor. So although its peak is only 4,205 metres (13,796 feet) above the sea level, it is the biggest mountain on the earth.

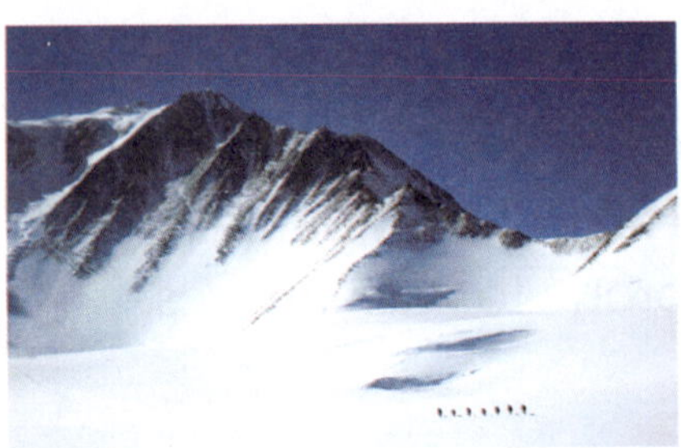

## Vinson Massif

Vinson Massif at about 4,897 metres (16, 067 feet), is the highest point of the Ellsworth range. It is located in Antarctica, which is a frozen continent.

## Mont Blanc

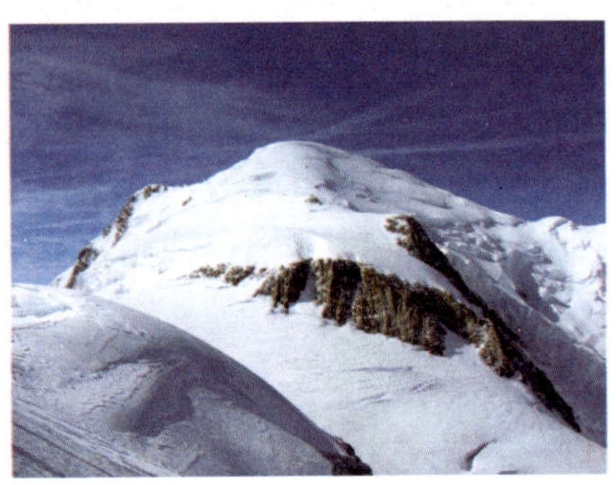

The European Alps were formed due to the movement of the African continent towards the north. The highest peak of these European Alps is the Mont Blanc, which rises about 4,808 metres (15,774 feet) above the sea level. This height is not fixed and continues to change as its summit is a dome of ice.

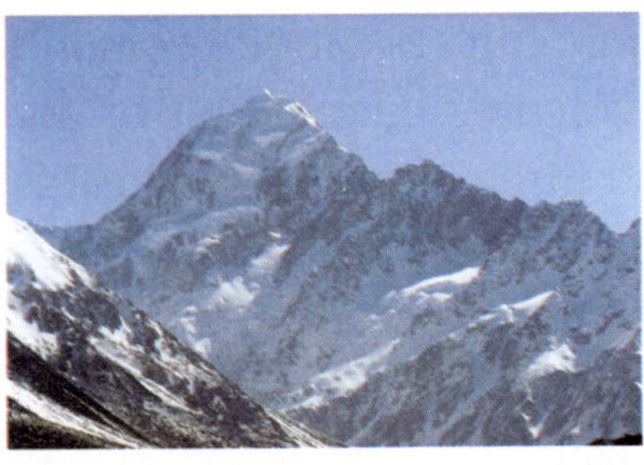

## Aoraki

Commonly known as *Mount Cook*, Aoraki is *New Zealand's highest peak.* Aoraki was 2,754 metres (12,317 feet) high, but after a landslide in 1991, its height was reduced by 10 m (33 ft).

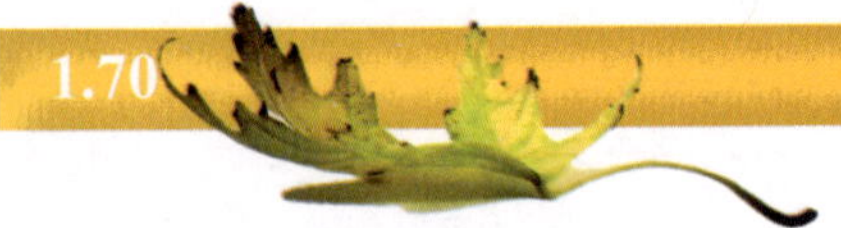

## Quick Facts

- More than 3,000 climbers have reached the summit of the Mount Everest.
- The snowy summit of Aconcagua is a part of the Earth's longest mountain range.
- Snow covers Mount McKinley all through the year.
- There is a 2.4-kilometre (1.5-mile) wide crater on Kibo's summit.
- The icy summit of Mont Blanc can rise to about 16 metres (52 feet) above its highest rocky peak.

Chapter - 6

# THE OCEANS

More than *two-thirds of the earth's surface is covered with oceans*. The average depth of the oceans is 3.8 kilometres (2.4 miles). These oceans are not merely pools of salty water. The ocean floors are the areas where the great plates of the earth's crust split apart or grind together, creating long, high **ridges** and deep **trenches** dotted with *volcanoes*. As a result of this, the oceans change their shape and size all the time.

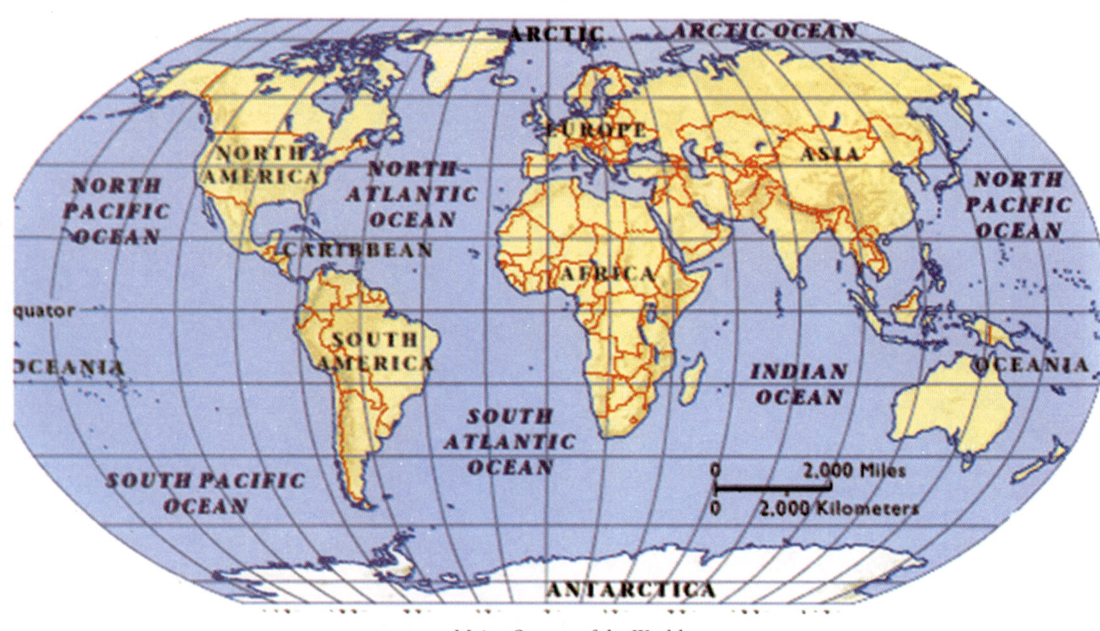


*Major Oceans of the World*

## The Pacific Ocean

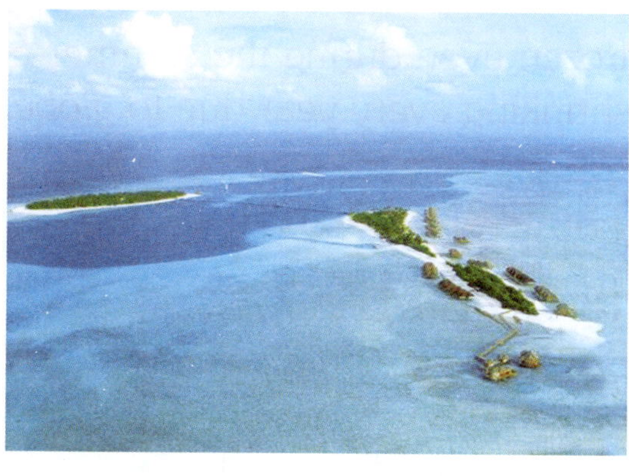

*Pacific Oceans*

As big as all the oceans put together, the Pacific Ocean is now shrinking. The reason behind this is that the edges of its floor are slipping into deep ocean trenches (a hollow space created in the ground for laying pipes or getting rid of accumulated water), such as the **Mariana Trench**.

## The Atlantic Ocean

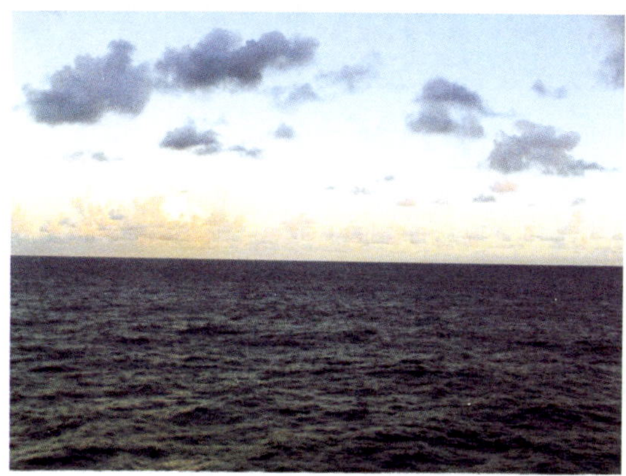

*Atlantic Ocean*

When North and South Africa broke away from Europe and Africa and moved towards the West, the Atlantic Ocean was formed. The ocean continues to grow as a new ocean floor is created at the *Mid-Atlantic Ridge*. The ridge breaks the surface in the north to form *Iceland*, with its *volcanoes* and *geysers*.

## The Arctic Ocean

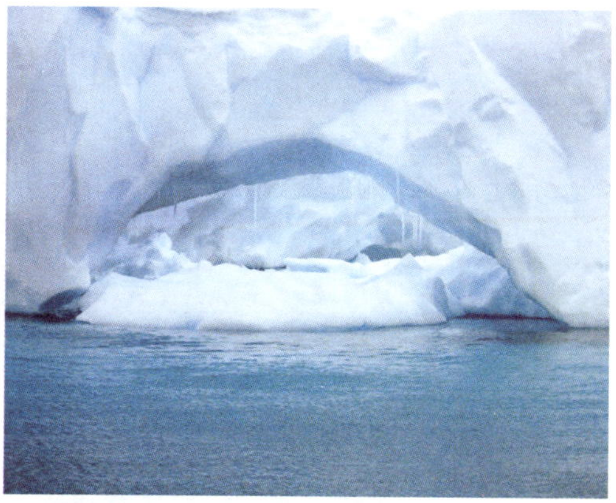

*Arctic Ocean*

The thick floating ice covers most of the Arctic Ocean. During spring, most of this ice melts, which allows the sunlight to reach the cold waters and helps the ocean life to grow and sustain itself. Though the sea near the North Pole stays

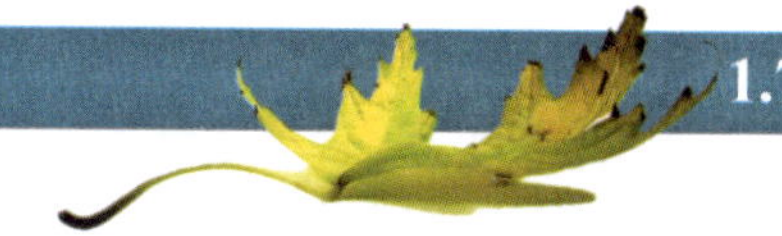

frozen even during the summer months, the area covered by ice is shrinking every year due to *global warming*.

## The Indian Ocean

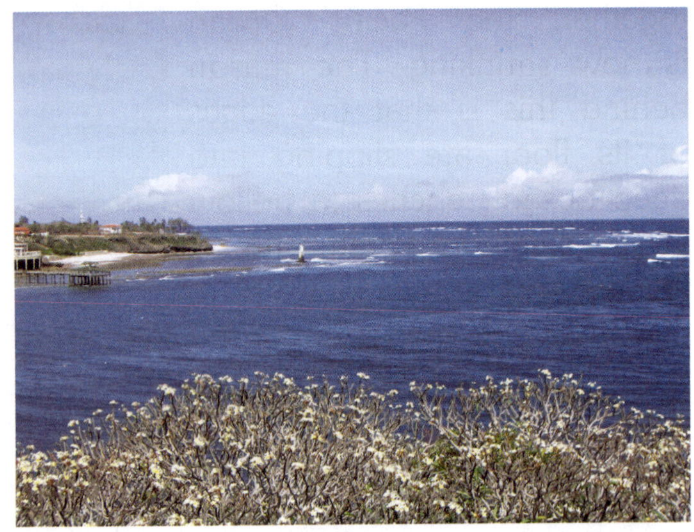

Indian Ocean

The Indian Ocean is basically a *tropical ocean*. It is very prone to *tsunamis*. It was last hit by a *tsunami in 2004*, which caused massive destruction on nearby coasts and various low-lying coral islands like the Maldives.

## The Southern Ocean

The Southern Ocean is also called the *Antarctic Ocean*. With no obvious northern boundaries, the Southern Ocean forms a ring of cold, stormy water around Antarctica. Ice covers a large area in winter, and the giant icebergs that break off the Antarctic glaciers and ice shelves sometimes drift well towards the north.

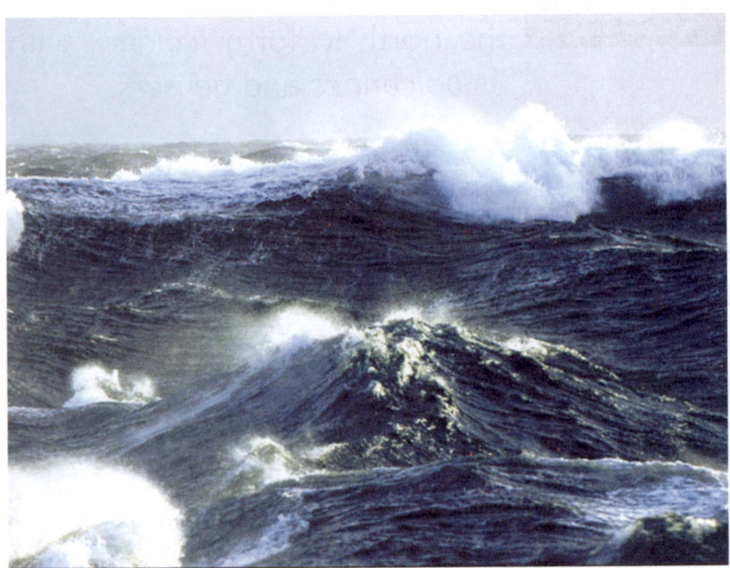

Antarctic Ocean

## Quick Facts

- The oceans cover around 71% of the surface of the earth and contain about 97% of all the water on the planet.
- The Pacific Ocean is the largest water body on the earth, and takes up one-third of the planet's surface. The name Pacific Ocean has an original meaning of 'peaceful sea'.
- Ocean tides are caused by the earth's rotation, while the moon and the sun's gravitational pull acts on the ocean water.
- The average depth of the oceans is more than 2.5 miles.
- The Antarctic ice sheet that forms and melts over the ocean each year is nearly twice the size of the United States.
- The world's oceans contain nearly 20 million tons of gold.

# Chapter - 7

# THE WEATHER

Without various weather systems, continents would only be barren deserts. Life would not exist in such a place. However, weather can also be very violent and cause a lot of death and destruction.

## Hailstones

Big *thunderclouds* have *upward currents*. These strong currents lift raindrops to a point, where the temperature is so low that they freeze. These ice pellets then fall down, but due to their light weight, they are again carried upwards. As a result, more ice freezes on these *pellets*, turning it into a big hailstone.

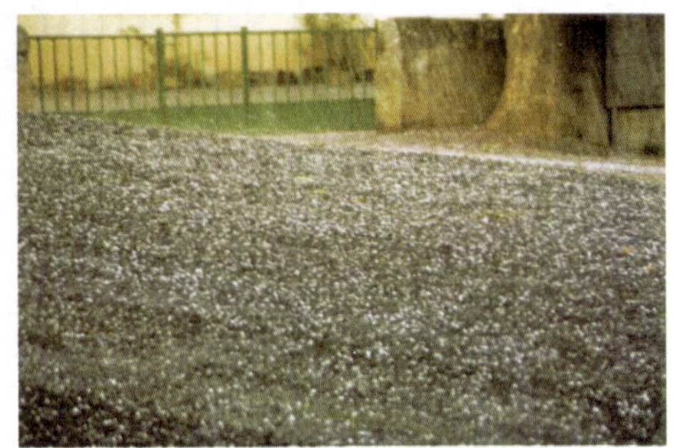

*Hailstones*

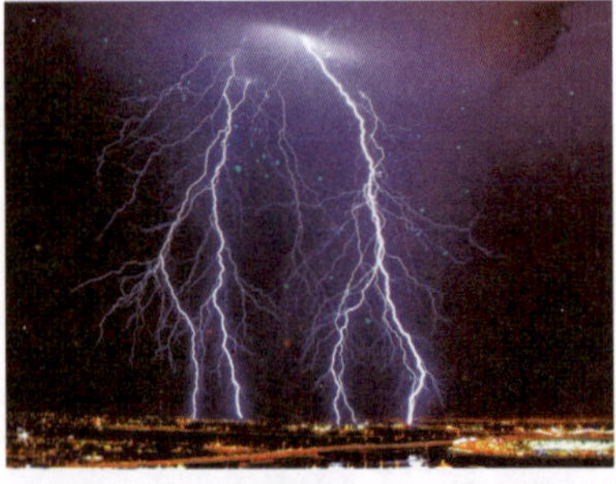

*Lightning*

## Lightning

When ice crystals get tossed around in a cloud, they charge the cloud with a lot of *electricity*. This charge is then released as *a bright spark of lightning*.

## Thunderstorms

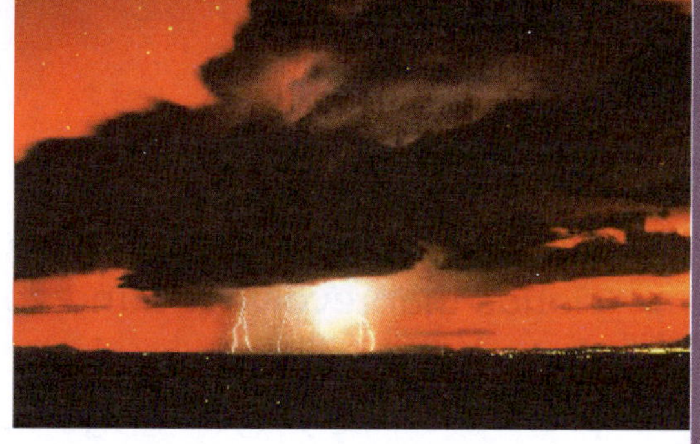

Thunderstorms

The sun's heat makes the water from oceans, seas, rivers, lakes and ponds *evaporate* (evaporation is the process of vaporisation of liquid either naturally or by boiling) and rise in the air. Here the water cools down and starts to form clouds. Some clouds go as high as 15 kilometres (9 miles) or even more. These clouds contain a lot of water, which is eventually released as a dramatic thunderstorm.

## Floods

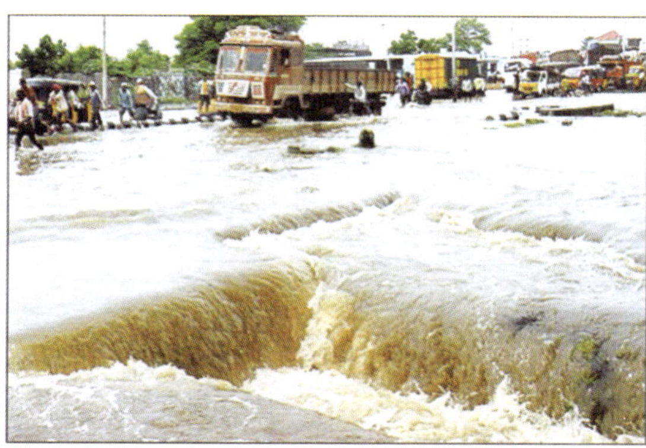

Floods

Heavy rainfall generally causes the rivers to overflow their banks. This results in *flooding* of the surrounding areas, especially the low-lying areas of land. This river water may also rush down valleys, causing *flash floods* that destroy everything in their way.

## Tornadoes

Rising moist, warm air forms *thunderclouds*. At times, this rising air develops into a tight, spinning *whirlpool of rising air*. This is known as a tornado. The speed of the wind inside the tornado can be more than 500 kilometres/hour (310 miles/hour), which can cause a lot of destruction.

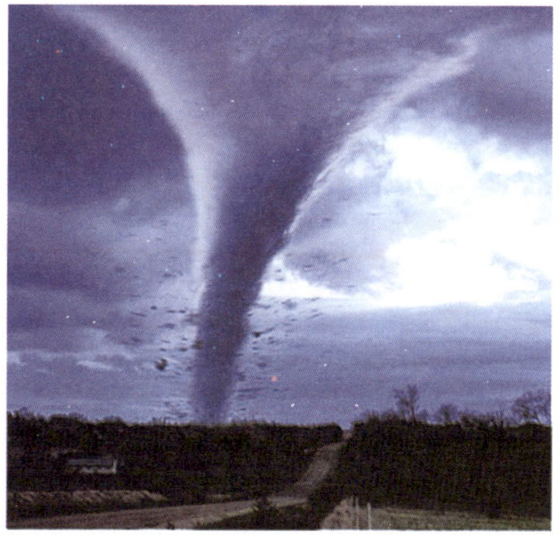

Tornadoes

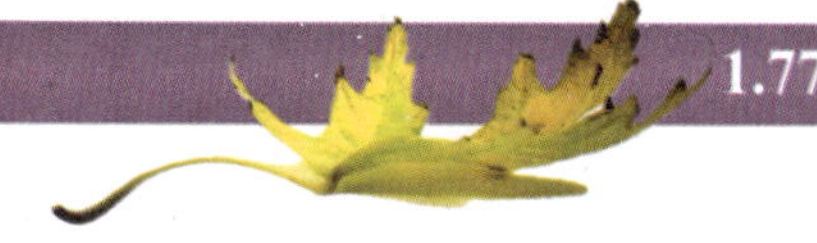

## Hurricanes

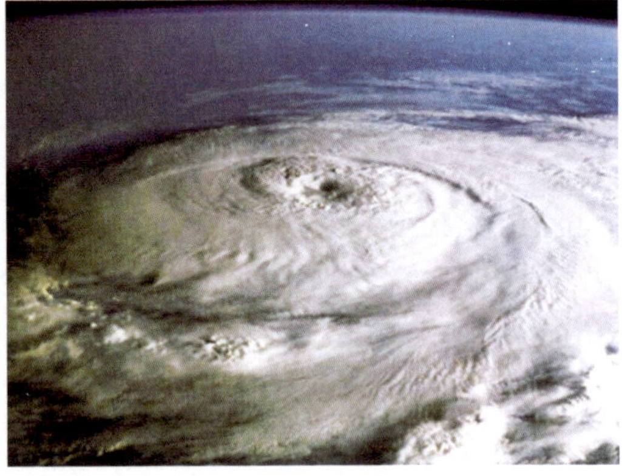

*Hurricanes*

Hurricanes are *enormous storm clouds* that revolve around zones that have extremely low air pressure. They generally occur over the tropical oceans due to intense heat in these areas. The winds in a hurricane move in a circular motion and can reach a speed of about 300 kilometres/hour (185 miles/hour). Hurricanes formed over the Pacific Ocean are known as *typhoons*.

### Quick Facts

- **The tornado is the most violent of all the earth's storms and the average lifespan of a tornado is less than 15 minutes.**
- **One lightning bolt has enough electricity to service around 200000 homes.**
- **The fastest speed by which a falling raindrop can hit you is 18 miles per hour.**
- **During a hurricane, 90 percent of the people die from drowning.**
- **The coldest temperature ever recorded was a negative 126.9 degrees Fahrenheit in Vostok Station, Antarctica.**
- **The typical lifetime of a small cloud is between 10 to 15 minutes.**

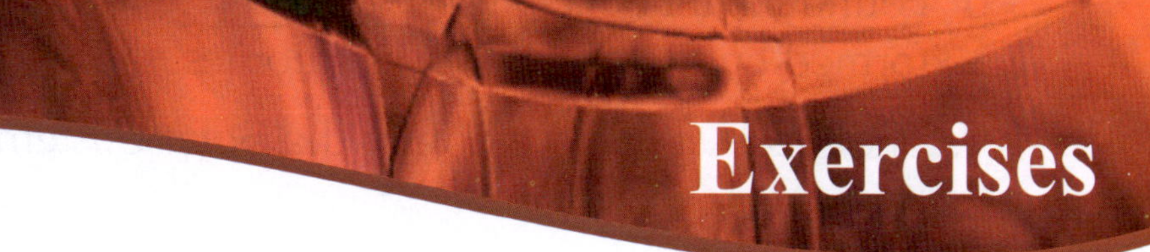

# Exercises

## I. Answer the following questions.

1. How was the Universe formed? What do you understand by the Big Bang? Describe it briefly with the help of a diagram.
2. What does the Universe consist of? Describe each part briefly.
3. What is a Galaxy and what are the different types of galaxies?
4. Explain the term, Milky Way.
5. What is a star and how long is the life of a star?
6. What are Nebulae? Explain with the help of an illustration.
7. What are Red Giants and White Dwarfs?
8. What are Star Clusters and what are the different types of Star Clusters?

## II. Fill in the blanks with suitable words.

1. The Sun is in the __________ of the Solar System and is one of the biggest stars in our galaxy.
2. Presently, there are ________ planets in the Solar System.
3. A _________ is made up of a lump of dirt and snow.
4. Russia launched the world's first artificial satellite, __________ into the Earth's orbit.
5. A solar eclipse occurs when the ________ is between the sun and the earth.

6. Found in Antarctica, the __________ Mountains have been formed by the __________ meteorites.
7. The most volcanic moon in the Solar System, __________ is very colourful.
8. The Earth was created about __________ years ago.
9. Earthquakes are recorded with the help of an instrument called the __________. It was devised by the American scientist, __________ in 1935.
10. __________ are the most destructive of all the geological features of the earth.

## III. Match the two columns correctly.

| | A | B |
|---|---|---|
| 1. | Mauna Kea | were formed due to the movement of the African continent towards the north. |
| 2. | The European Alps | is the biggest mountain on the earth. |
| 3. | The average depth of an ocean | rotation of the earth. |
| 4. | Ocean tides are caused by the | is more than 2.5 miles. |
| 5. | The oceans cover about | 71% of the surface of the earth. |
| 6. | One lightning bolt has | from drowning. |
| 7. | During a hurricane, 90 percent of the people die | coma and tail. |

8. We can see only a comet's | enough electricity to service about 200, 000 homes.

## IV. Multiple Choice Questions (MCQs)

1. The Solar System is not static, it is changing ________.

   a. Periodically  b. Constantly  c. Sometimes

2. Venus is the ________ planet in our sky and can sometimes be seen with the naked eye.

   a. Brightest  b. Dullest  c. Smallest

3. Saturn is the ________ planet of the Solar System

   a. Third largest  b. Second largest  c. Largest

4. The light from the sun reaches the earth in ________.

   a. Seven minutes  b. Nine minutes  c. Eight minutes

5. Till date, the biggest star found by the astronomers is called ________.

   a. Canis Majoris  b. The Sun  c. The Orion

# Glossary

**Asteroids:** Small solar bodies that orbit around the sun

**Astronomer:** A scientist who studies various bodies in the Universe

**Axis:** An imaginary line through the middle of anything

**Coma:** The head of the material which is formed when a comet passes closer to the sun than the orbit of Mars

**Diameter:** The length of a line that cuts across the centre of a circular object from one end to the other

**Equator:** An imaginary line that cuts through the centre of the earth

**Erosion:** The process of removal of the earth's topmost layer

**Evaporation:** The process of vaporisation of liquid, either naturally or by boiling

**Fault line:** A crack on the earth's surface usually caused by earthquakes

**Galaxy:** A very large group of stars which are held together by the force of gravity

**Gravity:** A force that causes objects to fall on the ground

**Impact craters:** Structures formed when a huge comet, asteroid or meteoroid crashes into a planet or a satellite

**Meteors:** Short-lived streaks of light of meteorites; also known as shooting stars

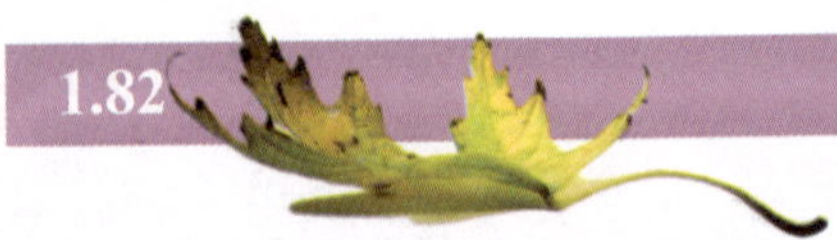

**Meteorites:** Rocky materials from the space that survive in the earth's atmosphere and land surface

**Meteoroids:** Rocky materials from the space that come close to the earth

**Nebulae:** Thick clouds of hydrogen gas in which stars are born

**Nuclear reaction:** The process of reacting various chemicals to produce nuclear energy

**Nucleus:** A lump of dirt and snow, which forms a nucleus; also known as dirty snowballs

**Oort cloud:** A vast sphere formed by all the comets together

**Seismograph:** An instrument that records earthquakes

**Spacewalk:** An astronaut's movement in the space outside the aircraft or the spacecraft

**Star cluster:** A group of stars that are close to each other in the space

**Stargazers:** People who study stars as an astronomer

**Telescope:** An instrument with lenses in it that help make distant objects look nearer

**Trench:** A hollow space created in the ground for laying pipes or getting rid of accumulated water

**Typhoons:** Hurricanes formed over the Pacific Ocean

**Weathering:** Breakdown of rocks, minerals and soils as a result of contact with the earth's atmosphere

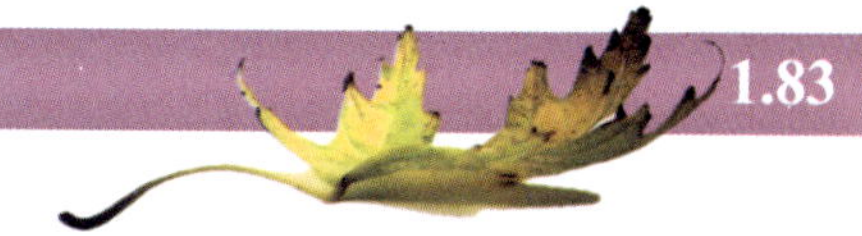

# ELECTRONICS

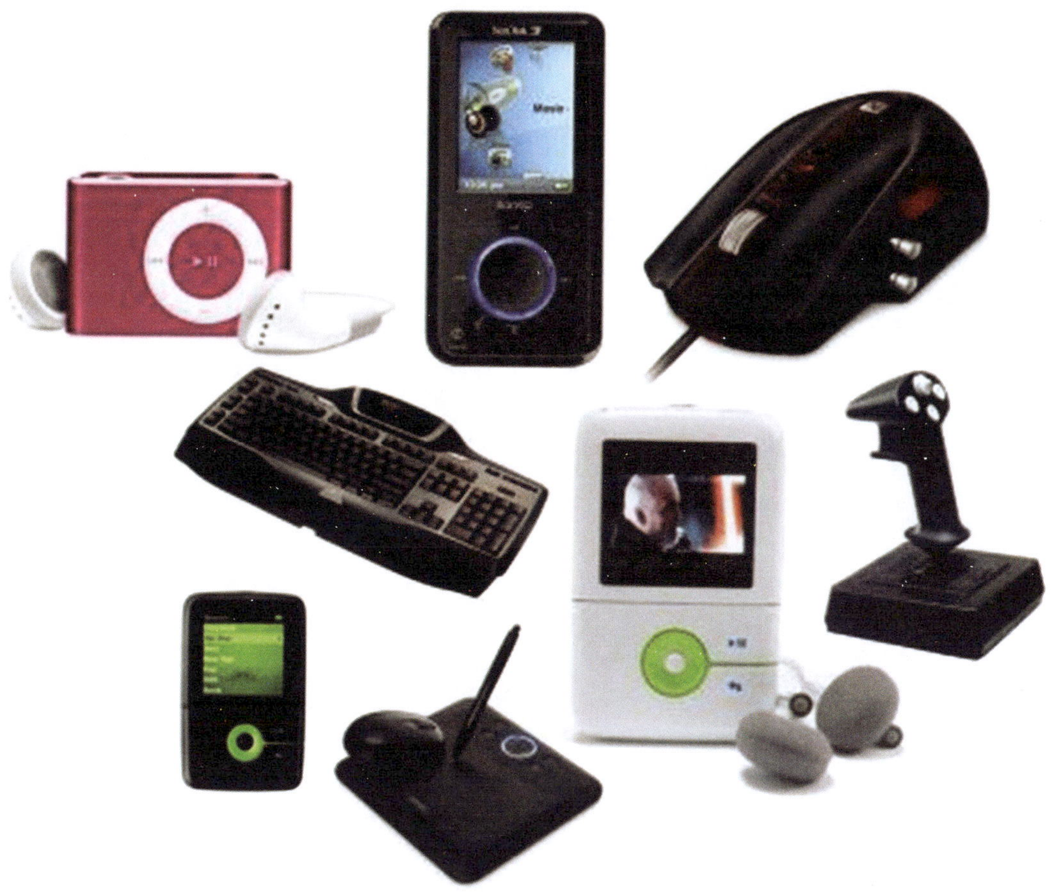

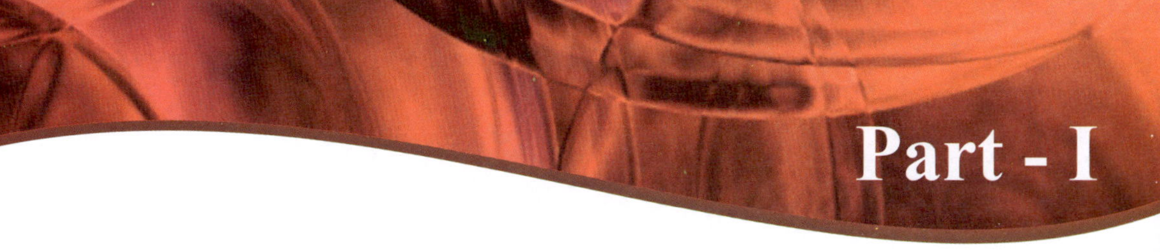

Part - I

# ELECTRONICS AND TRANSPORTATION

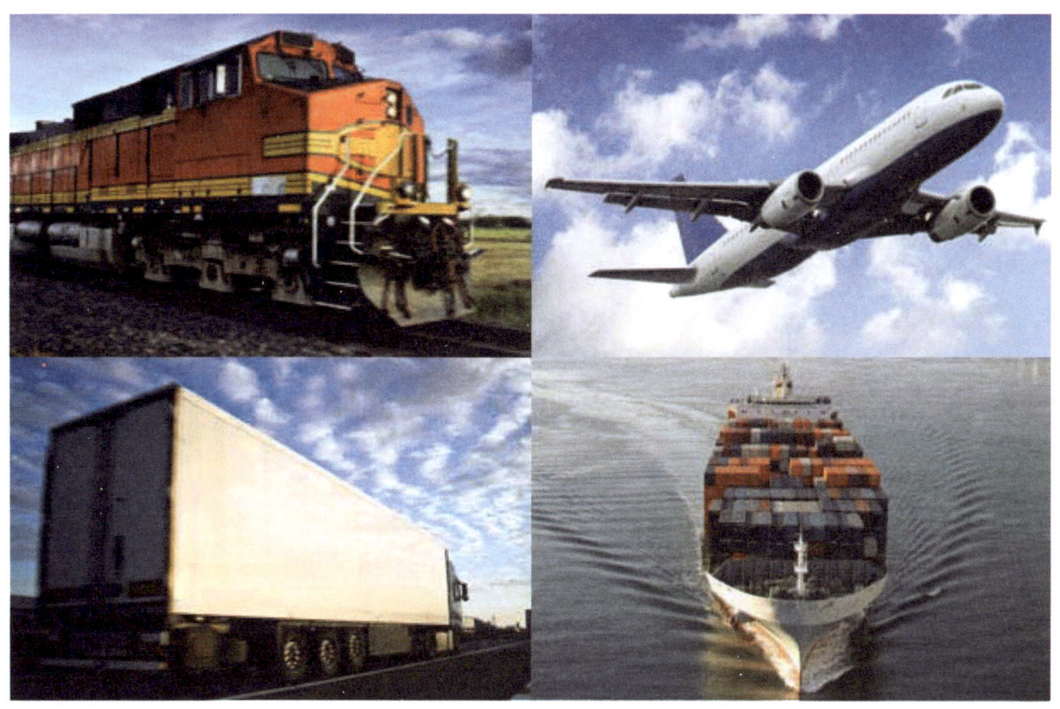

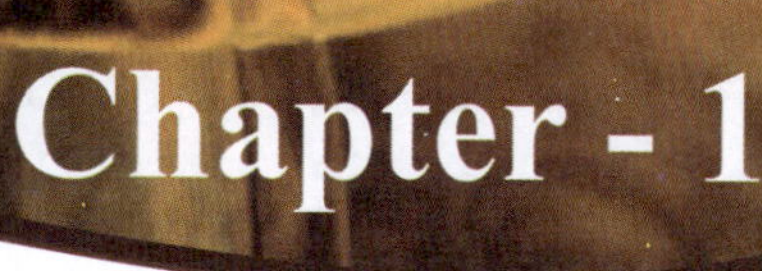


# INTRODUCTION TO TRANSPORTATION

## What is Transportation?

Movement of people, animals and things from one place to another is called *Transportation*.

The word, 'Transportation' is made up of two Latin words, *Trans* (meaning across) and *Port* (meaning to carry). So, transportation means carrying across people or things.

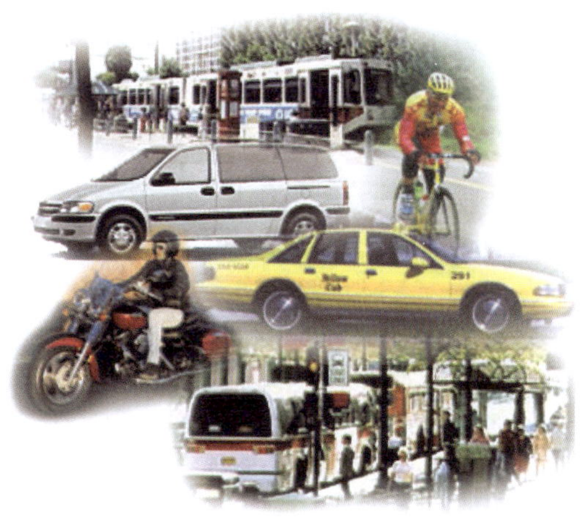

**Dictionary meaning:** *The action of transporting someone or something or the process of being transported is called Transportation.*

Vehicles used for this movement are called **Transport**.

There are *different types of transport for different modes of transportation*. For example:

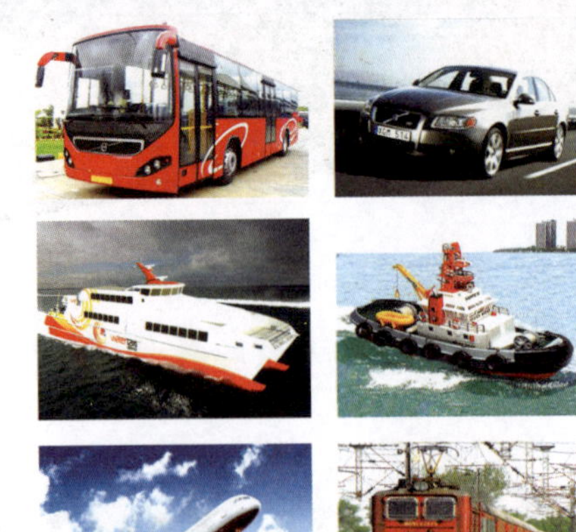

- Cars, buses, trucks, cycles and bikes run on roads.
- Boats, ferries, ships and cruises move on water.
- Aeroplanes, helicopters and jets fly in air.
- Passenger trains and carrier trains run on railway tracks.

These vehicles run on fuels like *petrol, diesel and CNG*. Some vehicles also run on *electricity*, such as the modern metro trains of today and the superfast electric trains like Rajdhani, Shatabdi, Mail trains and Express trains running across the country from one place to another.

## What is 'Fuel'?

Fuel is the substance which gives energy to a vehicle for running or moving from one place to another, in the same way as you give food to your body for working and living. Thus, petrol, *diesel, CNG and electricity* are in a way the food for a vehicle.

Small and light vehicles like cars, bikes and small motorboats need less fuel and generally, run on petrol. Nowadays, with the advent of *CNG or Compressed Natural Gas*, many large and heavy vehicles like trucks, buses, tempos, ferries, which need more fuel, run on diesel or CNG. However, there are also some small vehicles such as autorickshaws that run on CNG, which are a popular means of local public transport in cities and towns.

Bigger vehicles like *aeroplanes and ships* run on large amount of fuel. Some vehicles like *trains, metro and trams* run on electricity. There are a few trains which run on steam produced by burning coal. Vehicles like *cycles* and *cycle rickshaws* do not need any fuel to run; they run by *manual pedalling*.

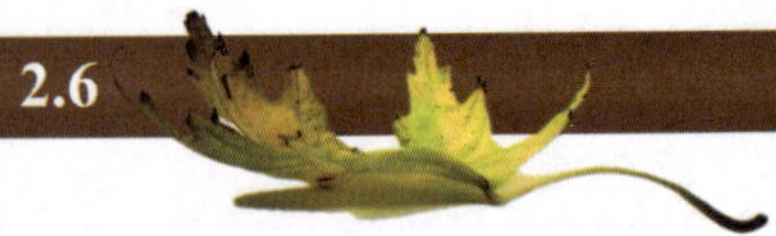

## Quick Facts

- There are more than 600 million cars in the world.
- In Delhi, public transport like buses and autorickshaws run on CNG.
- There are about 1,080,000 CNG vehicles in India.
- The first bus was set in motion in 1662, at the initiative of Blaise Pascal. The bus was then given a travel schedule, a fixed route, a charge carrier and of course, horses to put it in motion.
- In 1775, James Watt perfected the steam engine setting in motion a new era of public transportation. From then onwards, trains, buses, boats, etc., all began using the steam engine to 'improve' the life of the masses.
- In 1807, was invented the first steam vessel that carries passengers, even today in several parts of the world.
- In 1825, was built the world's first public railway between the cities of Stockton and Darlington.
- The first subway in the world was built in London in 1863.

# Chapter - 2

# ANCIENT TRANSPORTATION

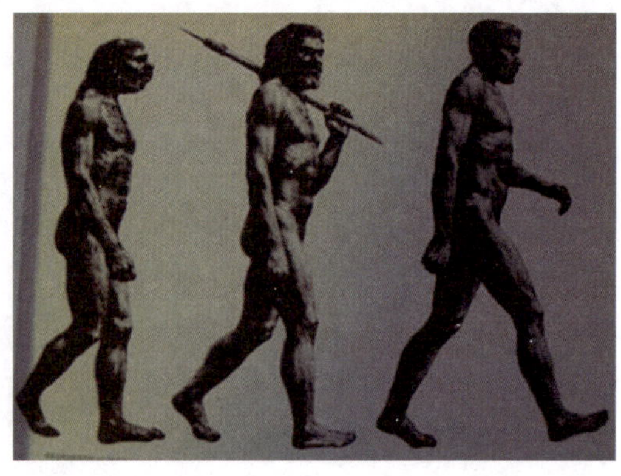

The term, 'ancient transportation' means the various means of transport used in the early age or ancient period.

During the early age, man used to walk to travel from one place to another or use animals like horses, camels, elephants, etc for transportation. This used to take a long time for one group of people to move from one settlement to another. After sometime, the early man started using stone and wood to make tools. With the use of these tools, he started making vehicles like carts and boats.

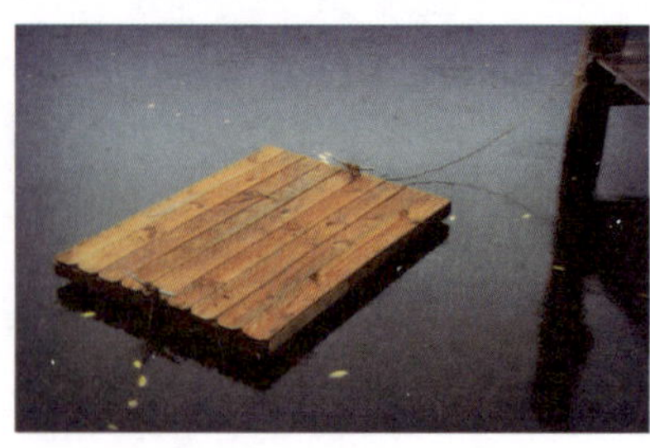

For crossing a water body like a lake or a river, he used to swim and travel. After sometime, the early man began using wood logs tied together by ropes to make rafts. In a few years, he also started making small boats from wood, for fishing and travelling.

## Dugout Canoe

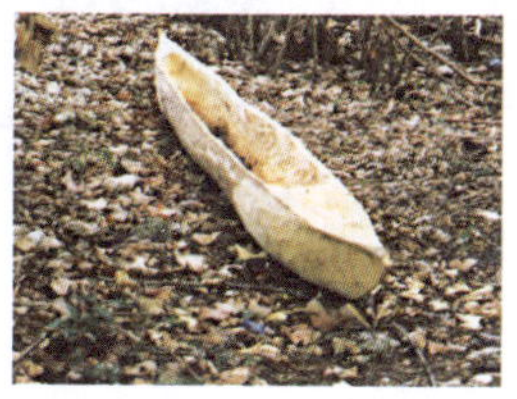

A dugout canoe is a boat which is made out of a tree trunk. It was first invented in the Stone Age by the early man. He used whole logs of tree trunks to make a dugout canoe with the help of fire and stone tools.

Dugout canoes were used mainly for carrying things, fishing and for carrying troops.

## Invention of Wheel

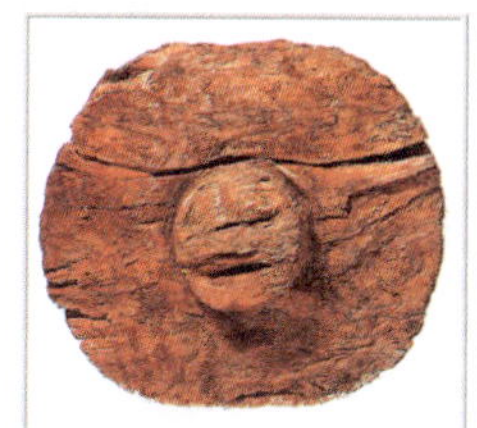

After the early man invented wheel, vehicles like carts pulled by animals were used for transportation. Animals like horse, ox, bullocks and camels were used to pull these carts. This was the best means of transportation as man could carry lots of things on carts and travel easily from one place to another.

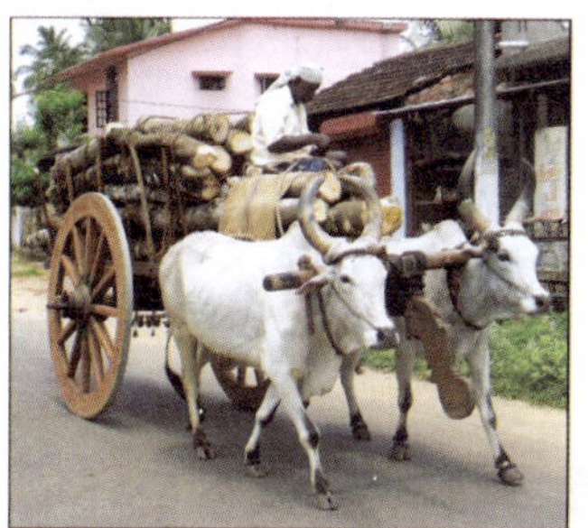

### Quick Facts

- **Man used wood and ropes to make animal carts. Later, he also put up a roof on the cart to shelter from rains, winds and heat.**
- **We can still find bullock carts in many small villages of our country.**
- **The first dugout canoe was invented in the Stone Age.**
- **The first wheeled cart was invented in 3500 BC.**
- **Horses were domesticated for transportation around 2000 BC.**

# MEDIEVAL TRANSPORTATION

The medieval means of transportation was used in the medieval age and it varied from region to region.

## Roads and Bridges

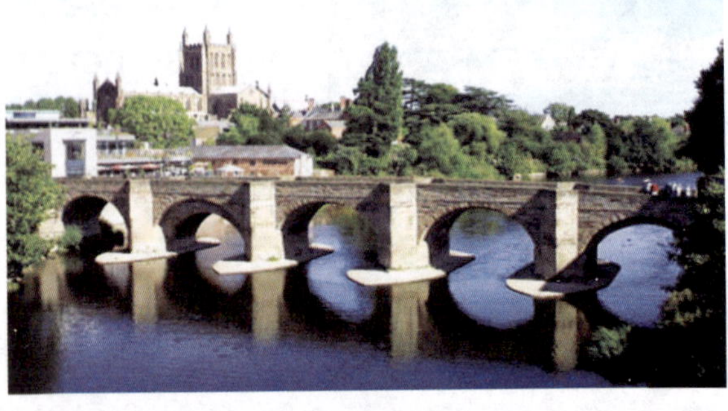

Roads came into existence with the advent of the medieval age. These roads were paved with stones and bricks. The development of paved roads made transportation easier for people.

Still, paved roads were not common everywhere. These were present only in the significant areas like city centres or shopping malls, trading areas, royal and government residences, etc.

The Roman road networks made during the Roman Empire are still famous.

In Europe, rivers were made crossable with the advent of bridges. These bridges were made up of stones and bricks and could bear light to medium load.

## Means of Transportation

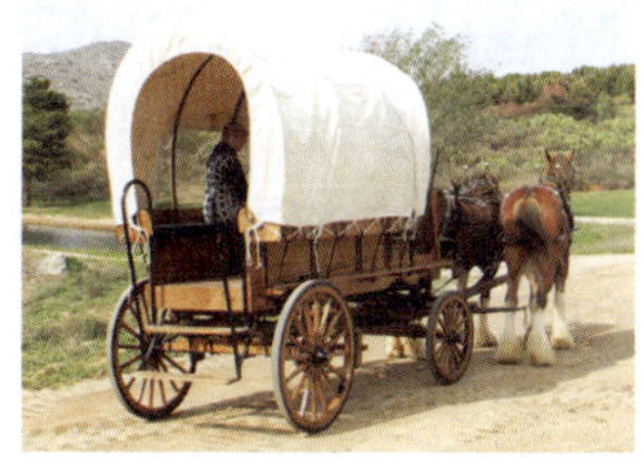

**Horses –** Horses were the main animals to be used for transportation. Rich people travelled by horses. Goods were transported by 'pack horses', i.e., horses with bags of goods on both their sides.

**Wagons –** Wagons were improved version of the wooden carts. They were mainly used to carry goods.

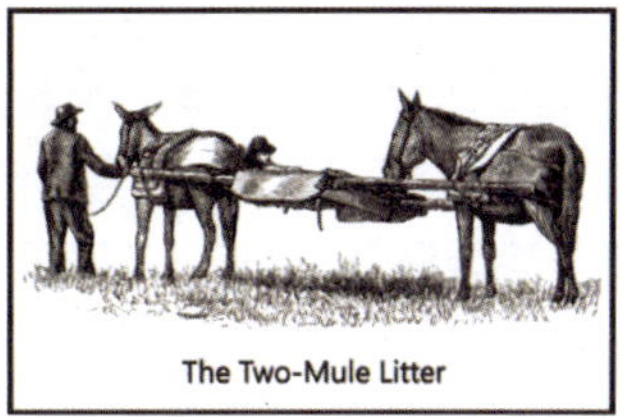

The Two-Mule Litter

**Litters –** Litters were wooden boxes big enough for a person to sit, supported by two parallel poles at two sides of the box. These poles were attached to two horses, one at front and the other at back. These horses were specially trained to walk at the same pace.

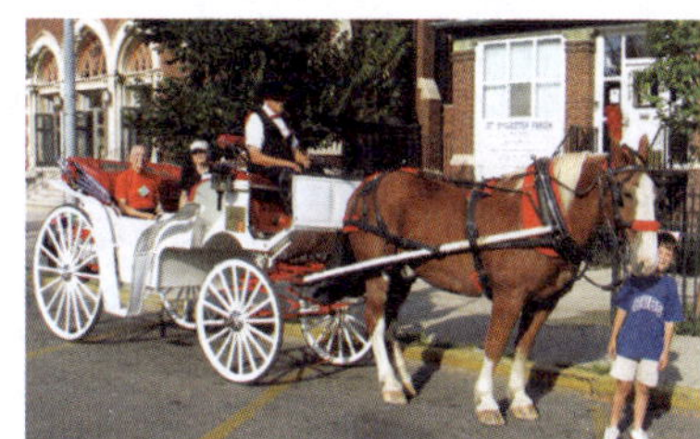

## Do You Know?

The first *President of India, Dr. Rajendra Prasad*, arrived in the *first Republic Day parade in a horse carriage*.

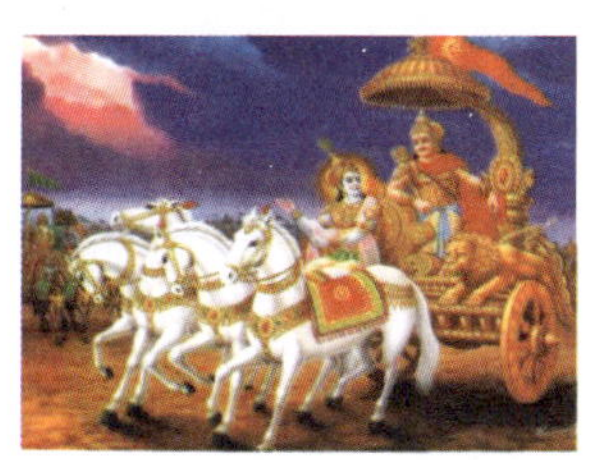

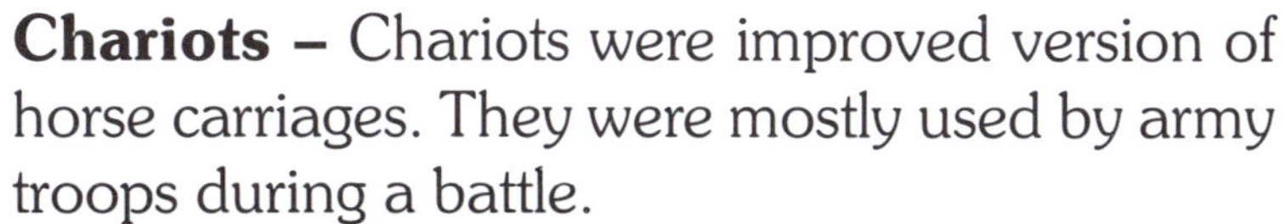

**Chariots –** Chariots were improved version of horse carriages. They were mostly used by army troops during a battle.

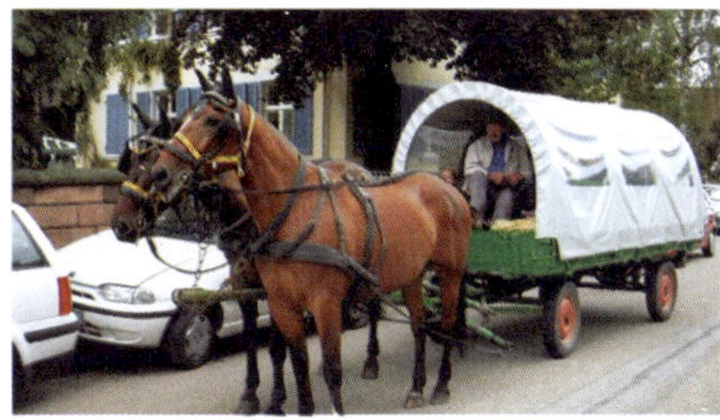

**Coach –** A coach is considered to be the first public transport. It was a covered carriage with a door and a window, in which four people could sit at the same time. It was attached to a horse and was driven by a coachman.

**Mast ships –** Ships were improved by erecting a cloth mast against a pole in it. Mast ships had better speed which made transportation easier and speedier.

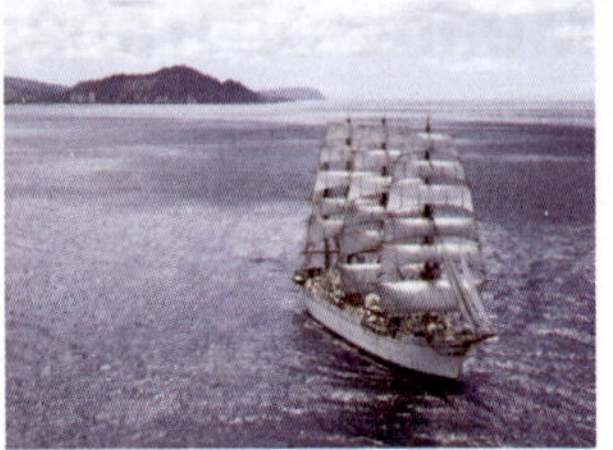

*Mast Ships*

## Quick Facts

- **A litter is very similar to a palanquin used in India to carry new brides. The only difference is that palanquins were carried by men on their shoulders.**
- **Carriages were horse driven wooden vehicles.**
- **The advent of the British saw trams being introduced in many cities including Mumbai and Kolkata. They are still in use in Kolkata and provide an emission-free means of transport.**

Chapter - 4

# TRANSPORTATION IN MODERN AGE

Modern Age transportation consists of vehicles like cars, buses, bikes, aeroplanes, trains, motorboats, etc.

## Invention of Automobile

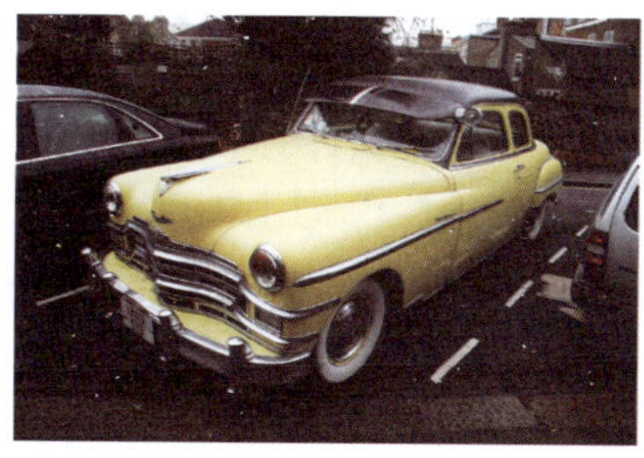

An automobile is a four-wheeled vehicle with a motor to run it. A car is a best example of an automobile.The word, *automobile* is derived from a mix of Greek word, *autos* which means 'self' and Latin word, *mobilis* which means 'movable'. Thus, automobile means a vehicle which can run on its own.

Following the development of an automobile, many other vehicles using similar technology have been brought on roads. Buses, trucks, bikes – all of them use their respective engines to run.

## Do You Know?

The term, *Car* is derived from the Latin word, *Carrus* or *Carrum* which means 'wheeled vehicle'.

# INVENTION OF AIRCRAFT

## An Aircraft

The Modern Age saw some of the greatest inventions in the field of air transportation. Prior to the modern age, there were some attempts to make humans fly in the air. These efforts resulted into – kites, hot-air balloons and gliders. But none of these attempts could be turned into successful means of transportation.

In the year, **1903, Wright brothers**, **Orville** and **Wilbur** demonstrated the first ever *airplane with a propeller*.

## Types of Aircraft

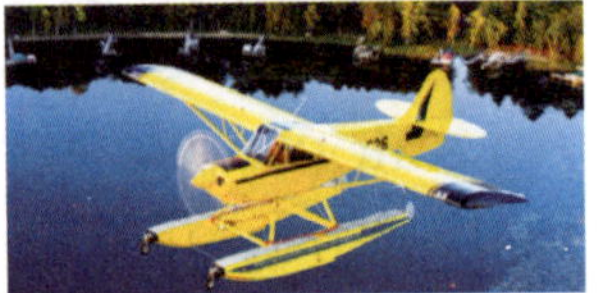

These were run on not so powerful engines and were not used much for commercial purposes.

**Subsonic–Boeing 747** is an example of *subsonic passenger and cargo plane*. It flies at 350-750 mph, just below the speed of sound, and is the most successful commercial aircraft.

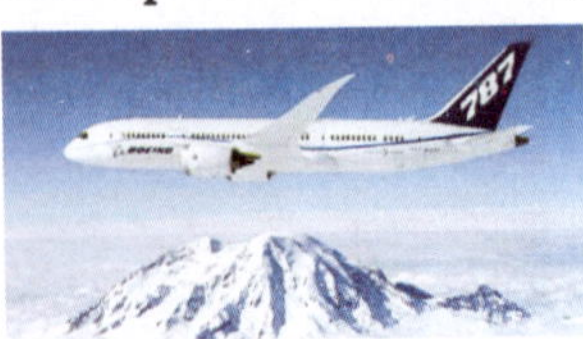


**Supersonic–A Concorde** is a good example of a supersonic plane which can fly at a speed of 750-3500 mph, i.e. five times the speed of sound.

**Hypersonic–A Space Shuttle** is an example of hypersonic plane. A hypersonic plane is attached to a rocket which flies 5-10 times more than the speed of sound, i.e., 3500-7000 mph.

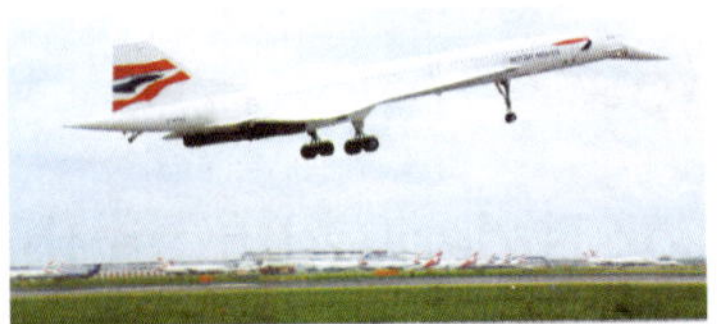

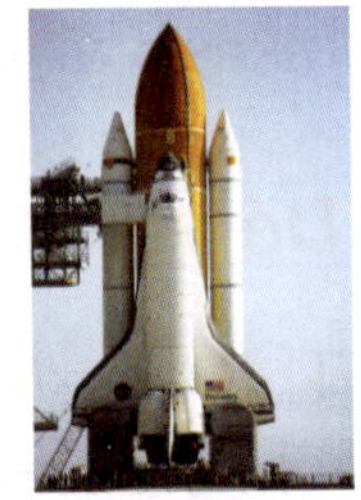

## Modern Railways

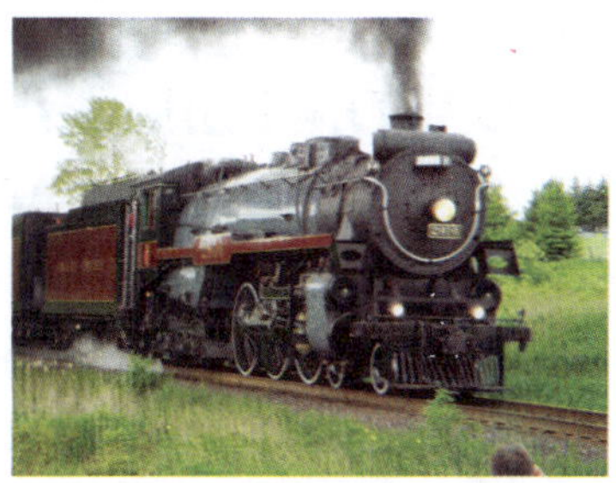

The modern system of railways was born in England in 1820s. Steam locomotives were the first modernised development or offering to the world. By 1900s, diesel engine locomotives came into use. By 1970, most of the railway networks in the world had started *diesel engine locomotives*.

## Do You Know?

The first steam engine was invented by **Thomas Newcomen**.

### Quick Facts

- **With the invention of wheels came the cycle which is still a very popular form of transport. In fact, in China it is the only form of conveyance for the common man. It does not require any fuel and therefore, does not harm the environment. It is an eco-friendly vehicle.**
- **The first invention that made transport truly fast was the invention of the steam engine. This led to the railways.**
- **The petrol engine soon changed the whole scene by making the motorcar possible. Today, of course, we have motorcycles, motorcars and diesel-run trucks.**
- **The first reliable motor vehicle to be used as a public transport was the electric train.**



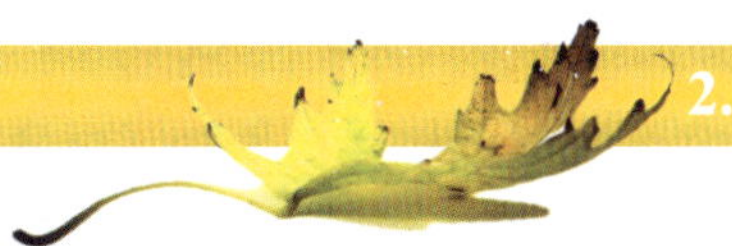

- The bulkiest of materials can easily be transported from one end of the country to the other end by means of trucks or by railways.
- Pipeline transport sends goods through a pipe, most commonly liquid and gases are sent, but pneumatic tubes can also send solid capsules using compressed air. For liquids/gases, any chemically stable liquid or gas can be sent through a pipeline. Short-distance systems exist for sewage, slurry, water and beer, while long-distance networks are used for petroleum and natural gas.
- Cable transport is a broad mode where vehicles are pulled by cables instead of an internal power source.
- Spaceflight is the transport out of the Earth's atmosphere into outer space by means of a spacecraft.
- The first modern rapid transit in India was the Kolkata Metro, with operations starting in 1984. The Delhi Metro in the capital city of New Delhi is the second conventional metro which began operations in 2002. The Namma Metro in Bengaluru is India's third operational rapid transit beginning operations in 2011. Currently, rapid transit systems have been deployed in these cities and more are under construction or in planning in several major cities of India.
- The Metro Systems under construction are the Mumbai Metro, the Rapid Metro Rail Gurgaon, the Jaipur Metro, the Chennai Metro, the Navi Mumbai Metro, the Hyderabad Metro, the Kochi Metro, etc.

Chapter - 5

# METHODS OF TRANSPORTATION

Transportation can be classified into three different categories depending upon the methods. The three methods of transportation are:

1. Manual
2. Animal-Powered
3. Mechanical

## Manual Transportation

Manual or human-powered transport is that type of transport where a man uses his muscle-power and energy to move the vehicle. These vehicles don't need any machine or scientific technology to run. Most of the vehicles used in the ancient times till the start of the modern age were manual/human-powered. Some of the examples of manual means of transport are:

- Hand carts
- Bicycles

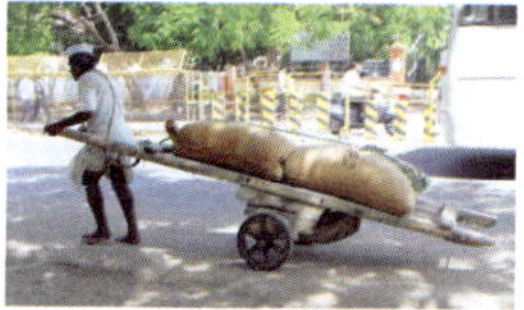

Hand Carts

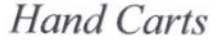

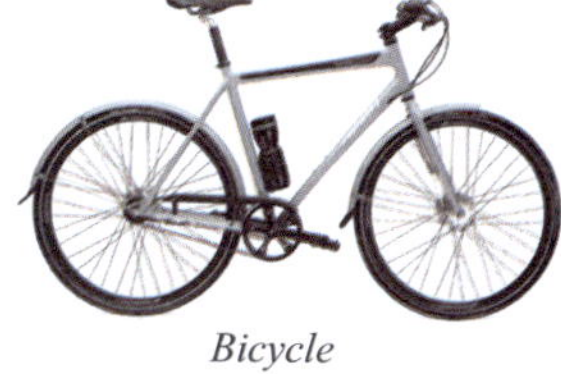

Bicycle

- Small boats
- Canoes
- Rafts

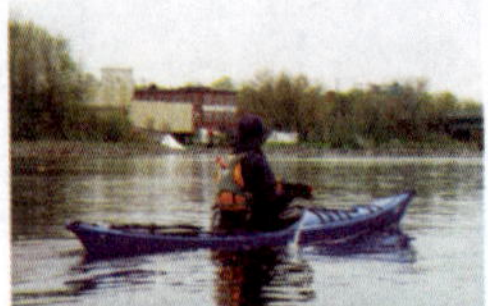
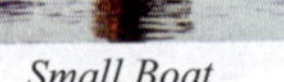
Small Boat

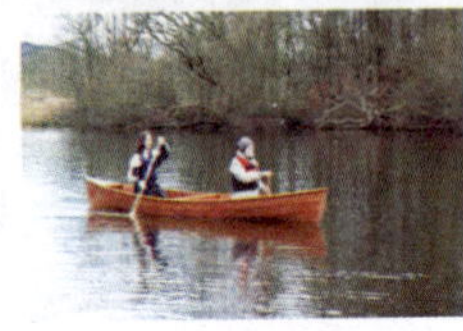
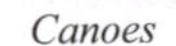
Canoes

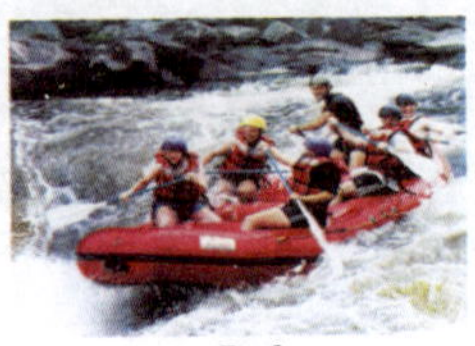
Raft

## Advantages of Manual Transport

- Low cost – These means of transport save money on fuel as well as on the maintenance.
- Environment-Friendly – These help in saving our environment because they don't run on pollution emitting fuels.

## Animal Powered Transportation

Animal-powered transport is that type of transport where animals are used to move the vehicles. Like manual means of transport, these vehicles also do not need any fuel or machine to run. These run by the muscle strength of animals like horses, camels, oxen.

Depending upon the region and the climate, different animals are used to power the vehicles. For example, in plains, animals like horses and oxen are used to pull the vehicles. In hilly terrains, mules and ponies are used while in snowy region, animals like yaks and big dogs are used for this purpose. Some examples of animal-powered transport are:

- Bullock cart
- Horse carriage
- Sleigh
- Sledge

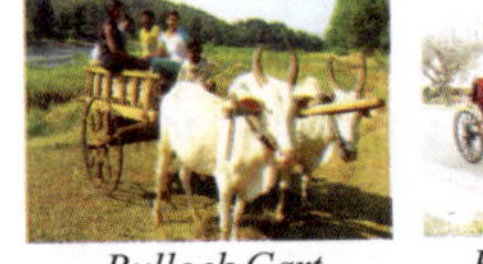
Bullock Cart

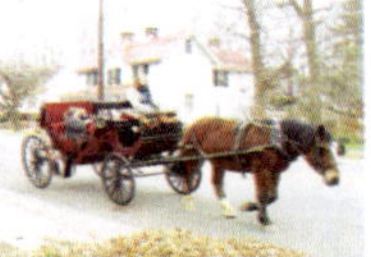
Horse Carriage

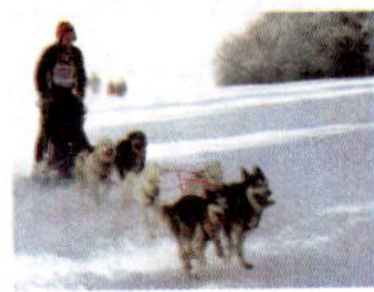
Sleigh

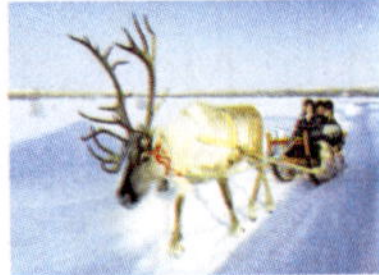
Sledge

Animal-powered transportation has same advantages as that of human powered, i.e., it saves cost as well as *environment pollution*. Moreover, it is better than human-powered transport as animals have better strength and capacity than humans.

## Mechanical Transportation

Mechanical transport is that type of transport which uses motors and machines to run. Unlike manual and animal-powered vehicles, these vehicles require fuel to generate energy for them to work. Today, most of the world uses mechanical transportation. Some examples are:

- Cars
- Buses
- Trains
- Aeroplanes

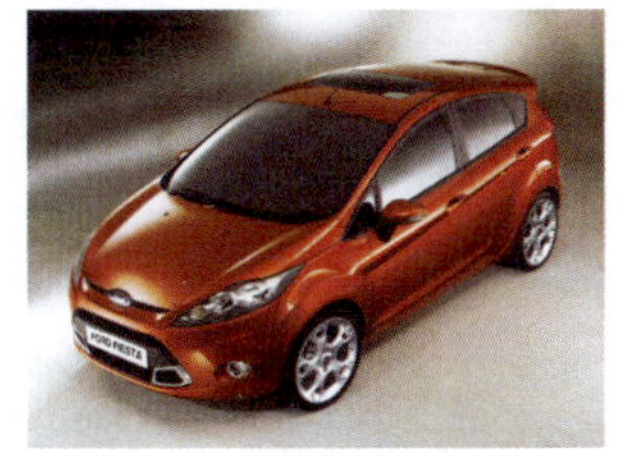

*Car*

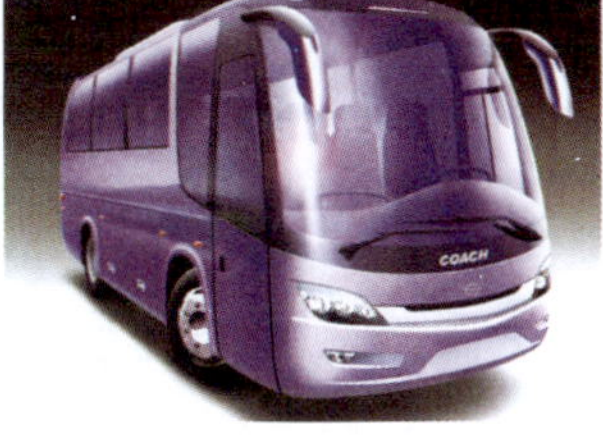

*Bus*

## Advantages of Mechanical Transportation:

**High speed –** These vehicles are very fast as compared to manual and animal-powered transportation as they are made using an advanced technology.

- **Saves time –**These means of transport save time during transportation because of their high speed.
- **Convenient –** They are very comfortable and convenient to use. For example: Most of them, nowadays, have air conditioners, comfortable seats, music systems, etc.

### Quick Facts

- **Pollution-emitting fuels are those which generate smoke after being used. Fuels like petrol, diesel and coal emit smoke which cause pollution in the atmosphere. We must make sure to use these fuels in small quantities to help keep our environment pollution-free.**

- Other environmental impacts of transport systems include traffic congestion and automobile-oriented urban sprawl, which can consume natural habitats and agricultural lands. By reducing transportation emissions globally, it is predicted that there will be significant positive effects on the Earth's air quality, acid rain, smog and climate change.
- The Rail based transit systems in India include the Suburban Railway (also referred as EMU/ DMU), Rail Rapid Transit or Metro Systems and Monorail.
- The present suburban railway services in India are limited and are operational only in Mumbai, Kolkata, Chennai, Delhi and MMTS Hyderabad.
- The first modern rapid transit in India was the Kolkata Metro, with operations starting in 1984. The Delhi Metro in the capital city of New Delhi is the second conventional metro which began operations in 2002.
- The Namma Metro in Bengaluru is India's third operational rapid transit beginning operations in 2011.

Chapter - 6

# TYPES OF TRANSPORTATION

Depending upon the usage of passenger transportation is divided into two categories:

- Public
- Private

## Public Transportation

Public transportation is that which is managed by government/ administrative authorities. Public transport, usually, runs on a fixed time and on a fixed route. For example, buses, trains, metros, taxis, autorickshaws, etc are all means of public transport.

In India, public transport, such as buses and autorickshaws come under the state control, whereas, taxis are owned by private companies. **The Indian Railways** is the biggest mode of public transport and is controlled by the Ministry of Railways under the Government of India.

## Do You Know?

Around 30 million people travel in the Indian Railways, daily.

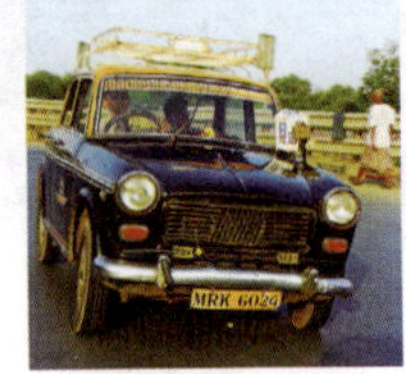


Public transportation is also a good source of revenue generation for the government.

## Advantages of Using Public Transport

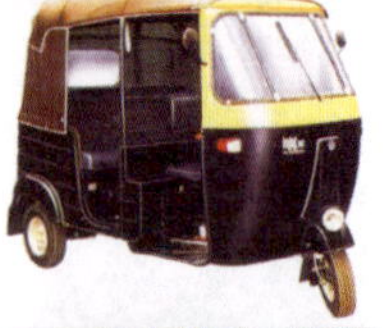

- Low cost
- Reduces pollution
- Reduces traffic jams
- Reduces usage of fuel
- Best means of transportation for people without private vehicles

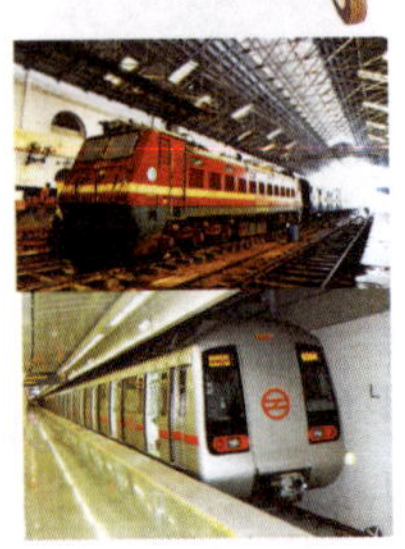

## Private Transportation

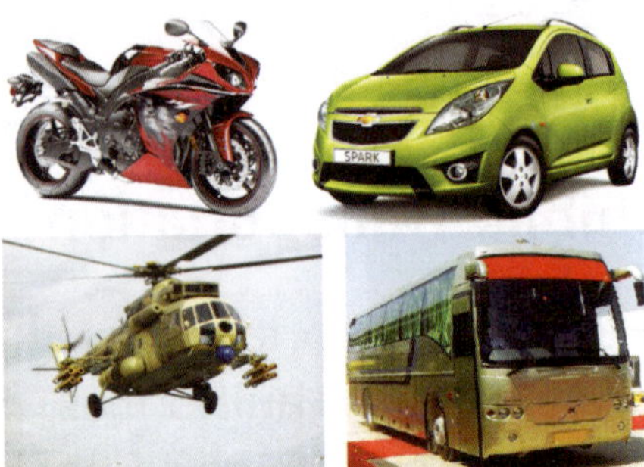


The private means of transport are those which are owned by individuals for their private use. For example, cars, bikes, cycles, private buses, vans, helicopters, etc. These are not available for the general public. People use private vehicles to meet their personal demands.

In India, out of the total registered vehicles per year, 95% are privately owned.

## Do You Know?

In Delhi, an average of *965 private vehicles* are registered daily.

Today, many privately owned cars are running on CNG and LPG like most of the public transport, in India. This helps in keeping a check on pollution and reducing individual carbon footprint.



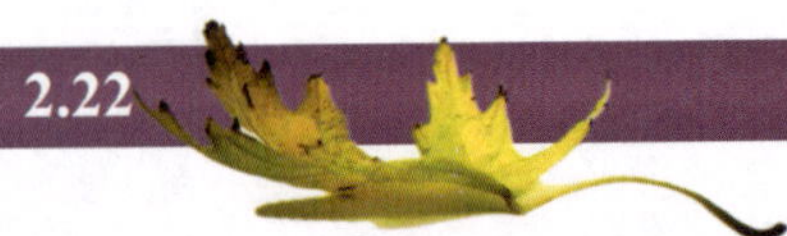

## Advantages of Using Private Transport

- It offers flexibility.
- It is not time bound and scheduled.
- It saves time unlike public transport.
- It provides privacy to the users.

## Means of Transportation

'Means of transport' is a term which describes and distinguishes different ways of transportation. There are *four different means of transportation – Roadways, Railways, Waterways and Airways*. For Roadways, the examples are cars, buses, vans, jeeps, trucks, etc. For Railways, the examples are Express trains, Mail trains, Metros, and for Waterways, we have ships, steamers, motorboats, cruises, boats, etc. For Airways, we have aeroplanes, jet planes, helicopters, etc.

### Quick Facts

- **Among all the metro cities of India, Delhi has the maximum number of vehicles (about 4.8 million) on road, followed by Bangalore or Bengaluru (around 3.1 million) and Chennai (about 3 million).**
- **India has one of the largest road networks in the world, aggregating to about 33 lakh kilometres at present. The country's road network consists of National Highways, State Highways, Expressways, major/other district roads and in villages — the rural roads.**
- **Approximately, 90 percent of the country's trade by volume (70 percent in terms of value) is moved**

through sea. India has the largest merchant shipping fleet among the developing countries.

- The coastline of India is dotted with 12 Major Ports and about 200 non-major ports. The Major Ports are under the purview of the central government, while the non-major ports come under the jurisdiction of the respective state governments.
- India has about 14,500 km of navigable inland waterways which comprise rivers, canals, backwaters, creeks.
- The Indian Railways is the largest railway system in the world under a single management.
- The Airports Authority of India (AAI) was created on 1st April 1995 by combining the International Airports Authority of India and the National Airports Authority.
- There are a total of about 20 international airports and many domestic airports.

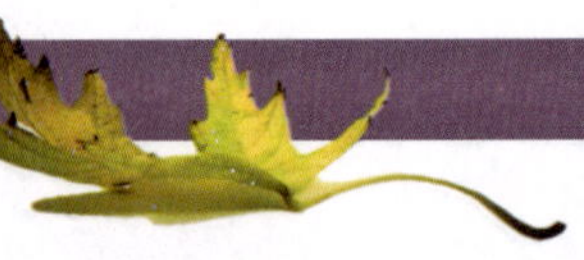

# THE ROADWAYS

A road is a route of travel which connects cities, towns and villages with each other. In a vast country like India, roads play a very important role in connecting the interior rural areas to urban regions.

## Stone-paved Roads

The stone-paved roads were first built in Mesopotamia and the Indus Valley Civilization.

## Construction of Roads

Modern roads are made up of materials like concrete, asphalt, stone and gravel. First of all, the process starts with removing obstacles in the route by blasting of huge rocks, digging of the earth, removal of stones and cutting trees. After the track is cleared, it is then paved with a mixture of asphalt, concrete, stone and gravel.

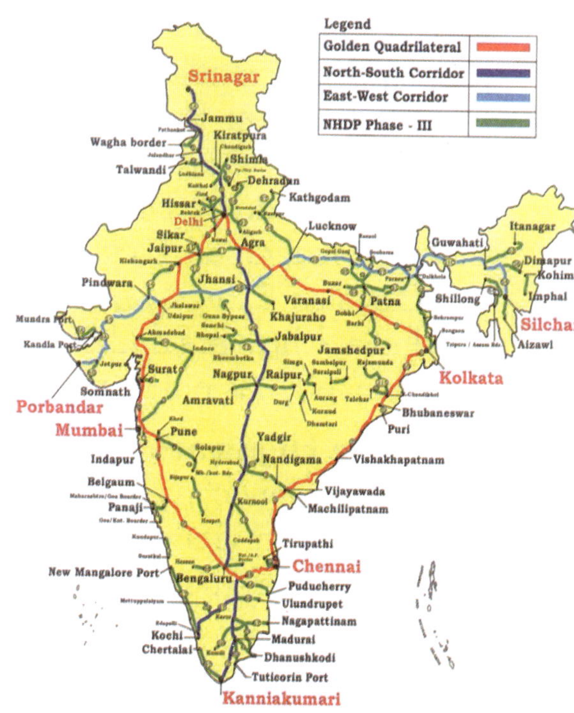

## Do You Know?

India has the third largest road network in the world with approximately 3,383,344 kilometres of roads.

**Types of Roads**

## The roads are classified into:

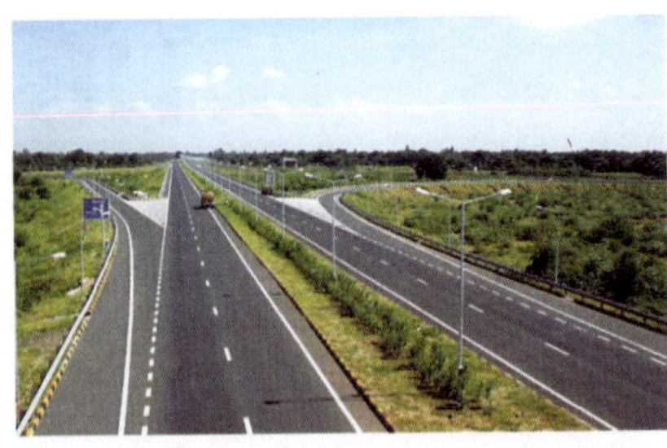

- **National Highways** – These are the roads connecting the state capitals and are financed by the central government.

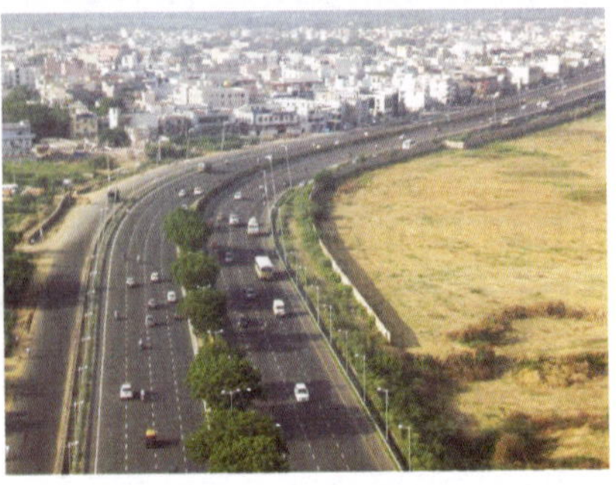

- **Expressways** – There are about 11 Super Expressways in India. They are the Ahmedabad Vadodara Expressway, the Mumbai-Pune Expressway, the Jaipur-Kishangarh Expressway, the Allahabad Bypass, the Ambala Chandigarh Expressway, the Chennai Bypass, the Delhi-Gurgaon Expressway, the Delhi-Noida Direct Flyway, the Hyderabad Elevated Expressway and the Hosur Road Elevated Expressway. There are many more expressways in India, which are under construction, or are already approved, but work has not started yet.

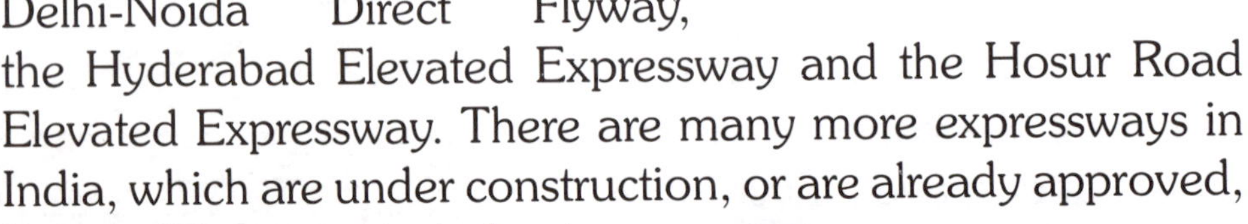

- **State Highways** – These are the roads connecting important cities in a state and are financed by the state government.

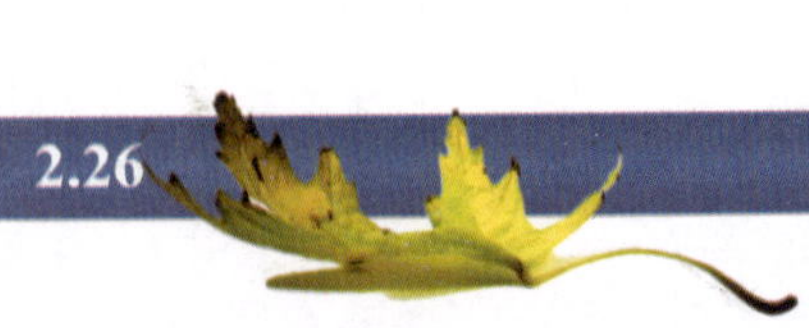

- **District Highways** – These are the roads connecting district headquarters and important towns in the district with state and national highways. They are funded by the Zila Parishads.

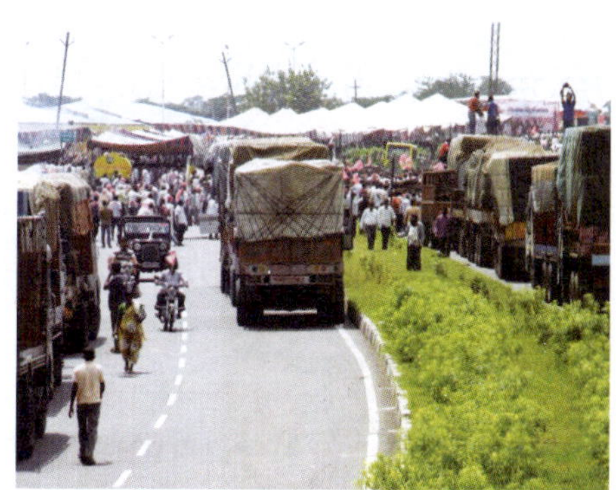

- **Village Roads** – These are the roads connecting several villages and to the nearest district highway. These are financed by the Village Panchayats.

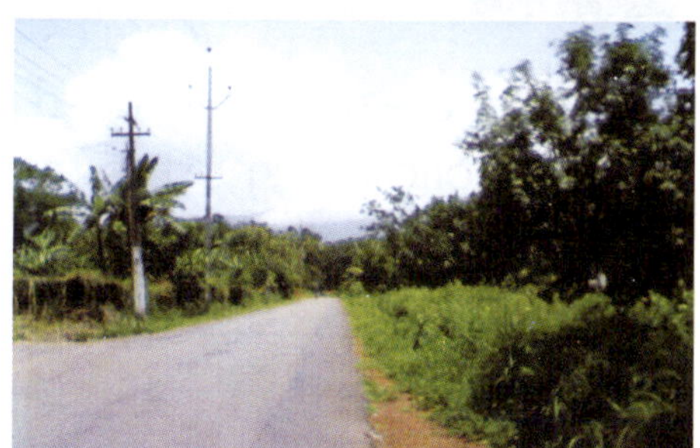

## Transportation

Vehicles running on roads constitute the roadways transportation. These are generally driven by automobiles with the use of motors.

Vehicles used for transportation purpose on roads are divided into:

- Passenger carrier vehicles
- Freight carrier vehicles

## Passenger Carrier Vehicles

Vehicles which are used to transport people are called passenger carriers. For example:

- Cycles
- Bikes
- Cars
- Autorickshaws
- Buses

People mostly drive cars, bikes and cycles for their private use. There are more than 51922 thousand two-wheelers and around 9451 thousand four-wheelers (as recorded in the year, 2004) running on roads in India.

Vehicles like buses and auto rickshaws are generally used for public transit. In India, public transport is the most widely used transport system.

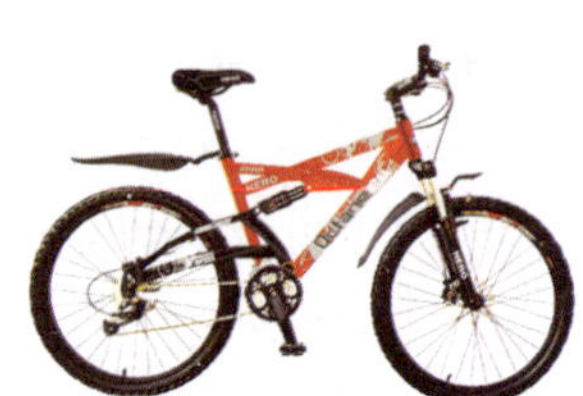

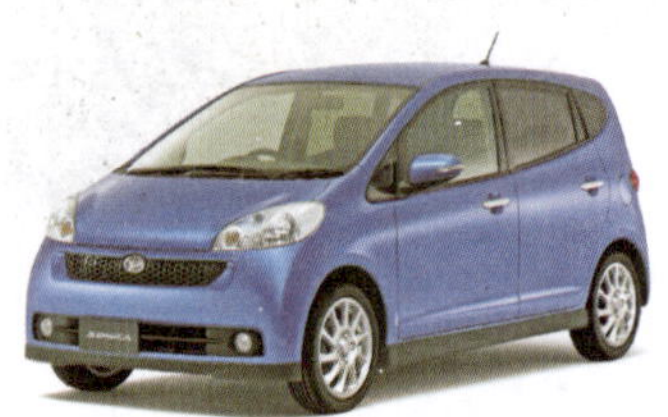

The term, 'Public Transit' is used to describe the transportation facility provided by the government to the people.

An automobile is a passenger vehicle run with the help of a motor.

## Freight Carrier Vehicles

Vehicles which are used to carry goods are called *freight carriers*. For example:

- Trucks
- Tempos
- Lorries
- Trailers

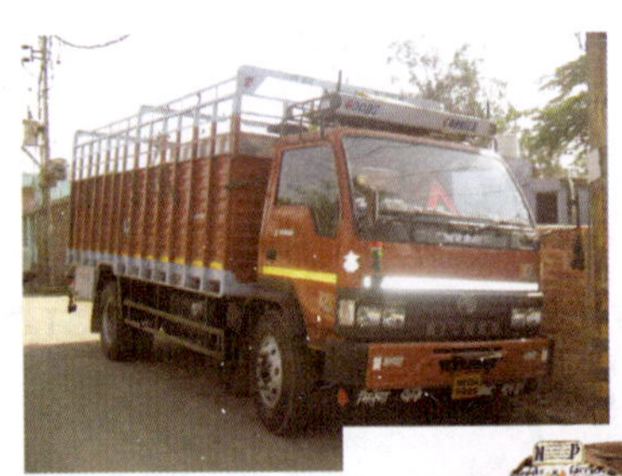

These vehicles save time and energy while transporting goods.

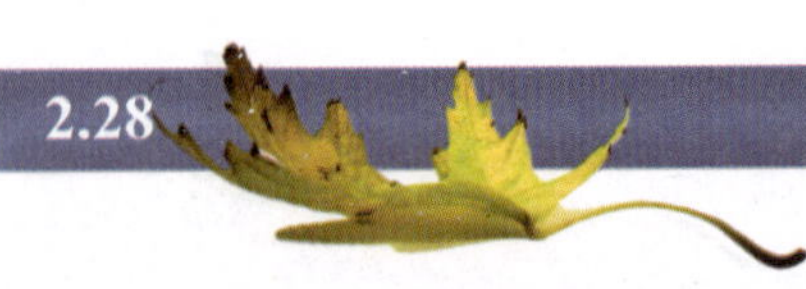

## Quick Facts

- In the year, 1897, the first car ran on the Indian roads.
- As long as 2600 km in length, the Grand Trunk Road (G.T. Road) is the busiest road in India.
- The Indian roads are left-hand-drive.
- Cars are right-hand-drive.
- Wearing seat belts is obligatory.
- Distances are mentioned in kilometres.

# THE RAILWAYS

The Railways constitute of a pair of parallel metal rail tracks fixed to sleepers, on which trains run carrying people and goods.

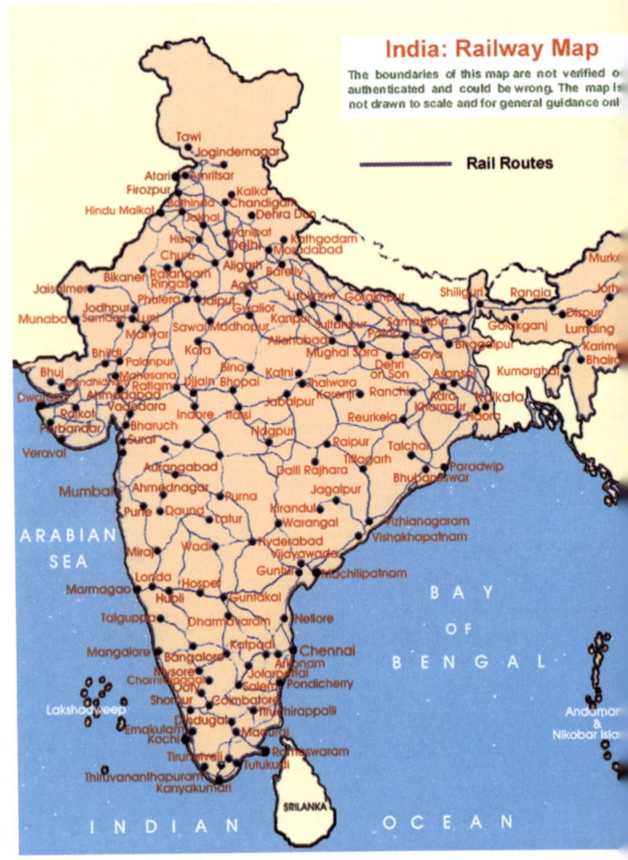


Unlike roadways, where vehicles run on prepared surfaces (roads), rail vehicles are guided to their way by the rail tracks. But, like roadways, the railways are also an important means of transportation.

## The Beginning of the Railways

*The first train in India ran from Bombay (now Mumbai) to Thane in the year, 1853.* The first locomotive was the **steam engine**, which used **coals** to create steam.

## Types of Rails

- **Broad gauge –** This is the most widely used railway track in India as most of the traffic is on the broad gauge.
- **Metre gauge –** This is used in the regions with less traffic.
- **Narrow gauge –** This is mostly used in the hilly terrain of the country.

## Types of Trains

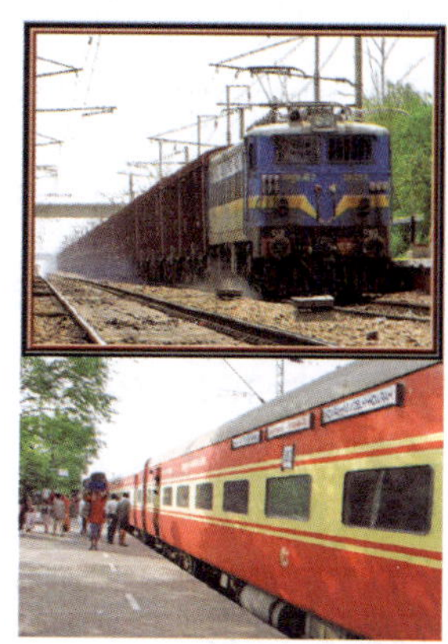

- **Passenger trains** – Trains which carry people are called passenger trains.
- **Goods trains** – Trains which carry goods, machines, vehicles, etc., from one place to another are called goods trains.

## Do You Know?

In India, trains carry more than *30 million people daily* and about *2.8 million tons of load daily* from one place to another.

## The Indian Railways

The Indian Railways rank **first** in *Asia* and **fourth** in the *world*. Today, more than *11000 trains* run in the railway network of our country. The length of the Indian Railways is more than **111,599 km**.

The Indian Railways is divided into the following zones:

1. Central Railways
2. Northern Railways
3. North-eastern Railways
4. North-western Railways
5. North-central Railways

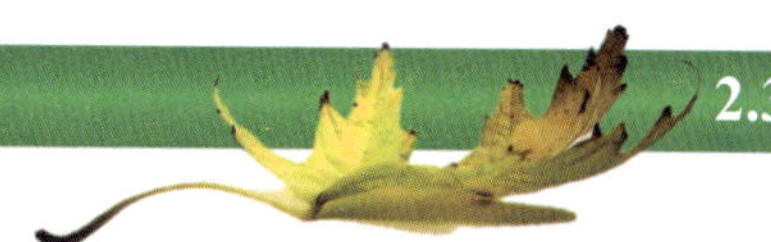

6. North-east Frontier Railways
7. Eastern Railways
8. East-central Railways
9. East coast Railways
10. Western Railways
11. West-central Railways
12. Southern Railways
13. South-central Railways
14. South-western Railways
15. South-east central Railways
16. South-eastern Railways

Some of the significant rail routes which connect important cities of India are:

1. Delhi to Mumbai
2. Delhi to Kalka
3. Delhi to Chennai
4. Delhi to Aurangabad
5. Mumbai to Amritsar
6. Mumbai to Bangalore or Bengaluru
7. Mumbai to Vijayawada
8. Saharanpur to Varanasi
9. Lucknow to Guwahati
10. Kolkata to Chennai
11. Chennai to Jammu
12. Delhi to Kolkata

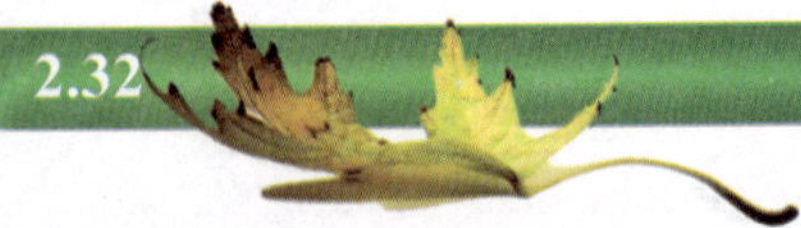

## Quick Facts

- The word, 'railway' was first coined in the year, 1776.
- The first railway was opened in 1825. It was the Stockton & Darlington Railroad, which was opened on September 27, 1825.
- The Indian Railways is the lifeline of the average Indians. The Indian Railways have continued to exist since more than 150 years.
- The Indian Railways employ more than 1.6 million people, thus becoming the largest utility employer in the world.
- There are more than 7,500 railway stations in India.
- There is a fleet of about 7800 locomotives in India and around 40,000 coaches.
- The establishment of the National Rail Museum took place in 1977.
- In 1986, the first Computerised Reservation System began in New Delhi.
- Sri Venkatanarasimharajuvariapeta in Tamil Nadu is the longest station name of India.
- The first electric train came into force on February 3, 1925 between Bombay VT (Mumbai) and Kurla.

# THE AIRWAYS

The Airways are the fastest means of transportation in the world today. It consists of winged crafts like aeroplanes, helicopters, etc. This means of transportation requires an *airbase* and a *runway* from where the planes take off as well as land on. Because of the huge size of the aircraft and the airbase, it becomes the costliest means of transportation.

Unlike other means of transportation, the airways are not divided into passenger and goods carriers. Here, big planes like *Airbuses* and *Boeings* also carry freights/goods along with the passengers.

Helicopters carry a maximum of 2-3 people at once, whereas a Boeing carries around 400-500 people.

The Airways have two branches:

- **International Transportation** – Planes carrying passengers as well as goods from one country to another come under international transportation. Air services like the Air India, Jet Airways, British Airways, etc provide international travel to people.

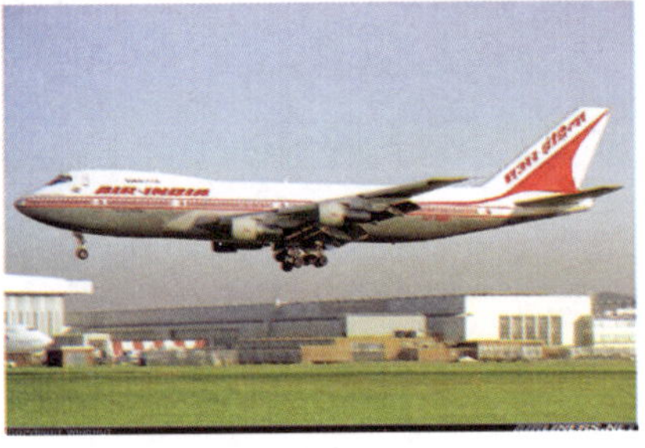

- **Domestic Transportation** – Planes carrying passengers as well as goods within a country, from one region to another, come under domestic transportation. Services like the Indian *Airlines, Spicejet, IndiGo* are domestic airlines.

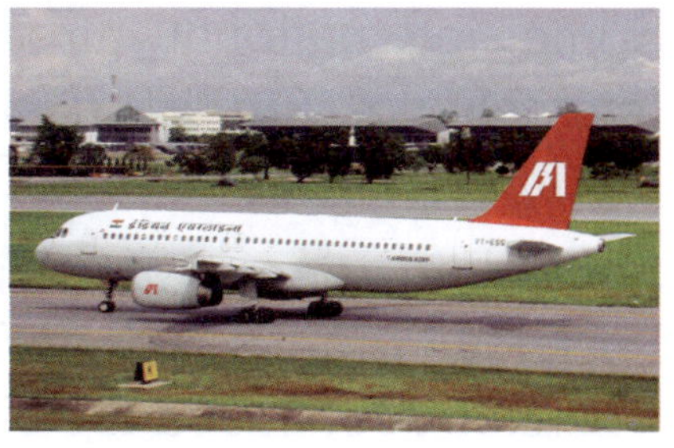

These planes are run publicly as well as privately.

The **Indian Public Sector Airways** include the **Air India** and the **Indian Airlines**. These are managed by the government and are the official airlines of India.

**The Private Airlines** include the **Jet Airways**, the **Kingfisher**, the **Spicejet**, etc. These are run by private companies. The private airlines

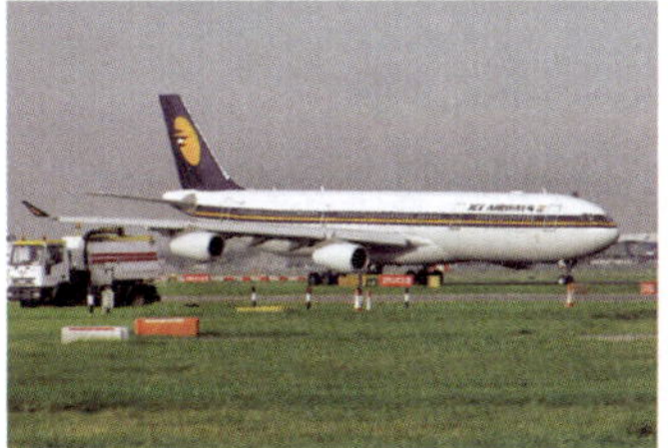

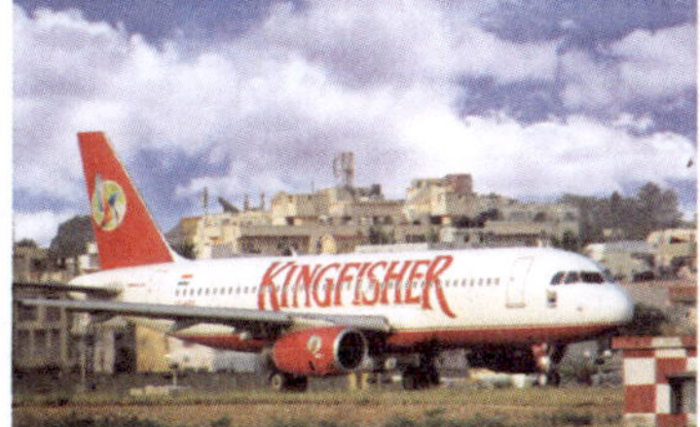


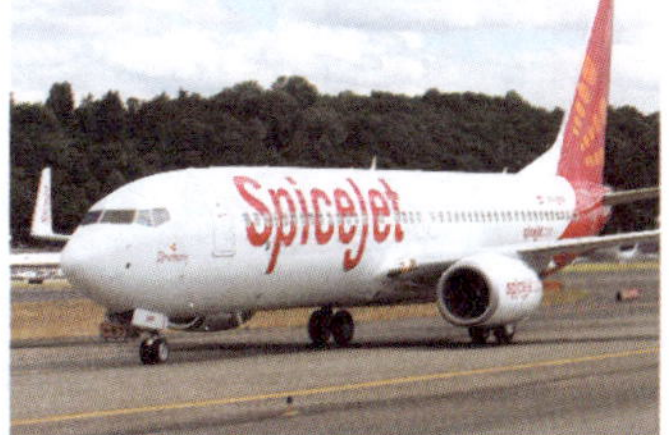


are more profit-oriented, and they also provide more flexibility. They also provide private **jet planes** as well as **helicopters** to important and rich people.

## Airports

Airports are the most important aspect of airway travel as these are the places, where people gather to board and de-board a plane. Airports include runways for planes to take-off as well as land.

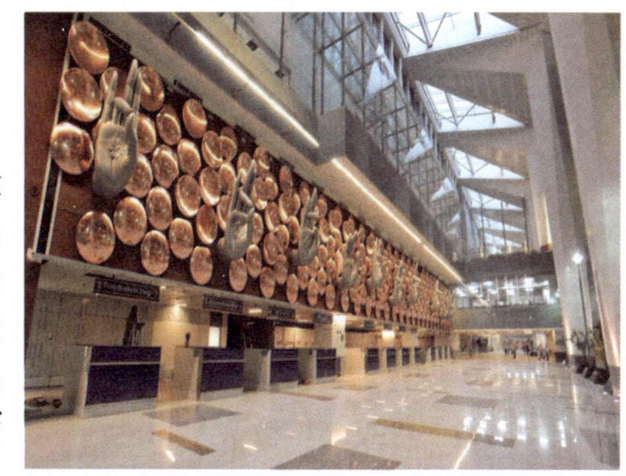

*Indira Gandhi International Airport*

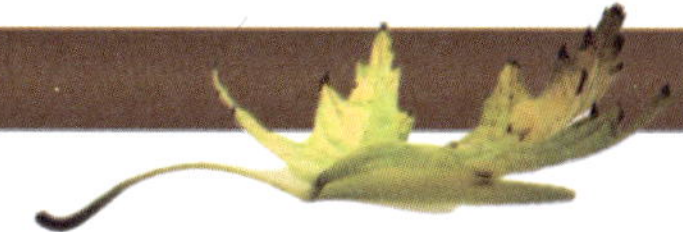

Some international airports of India are the *Indira Gandhi International Airport (New Delhi), Chhatrapati Shivaji Airport (Mumbai), Netaji Subhas Chandra Bose Airport (Kolkata)*, etc.

Some domestic airports of India are in cities like New Delhi, Mumbai, Lucknow, Amritsar, Chandigarh, Kolkata, Bangalore (Bengaluru), Chennai, Ahmedabad, etc.

## Quick Facts

- **Air India Limited is the major international carrier of the country.**
- **The Indian Airlines is the major domestic air carrier of the country. It operates to 57 domestic stations (including Alliance Air operations) and 17 international stations in 14 countries.**
- **The Pawan Hans Helicopters Limited has been providing helicopter support services to the petroleum sector including the ONGC, the Oil India Limited and the Hardy Exploration at Chennai. Apart from these, it also provides services to certain state governments and public sector undertakings and in the north-eastern states.**
- **The development of airports is no longer solely under the public sector; instead private participation is allowed and encouraged. An International green field airport has been developed in Cochin, Kerala, with contributions from NRIs and loans from financial institutions.**

# THE WATERWAYS

A waterway is an integral means of transportation in a country like ours which is a **peninsula** and where so many rivers flow across the land.

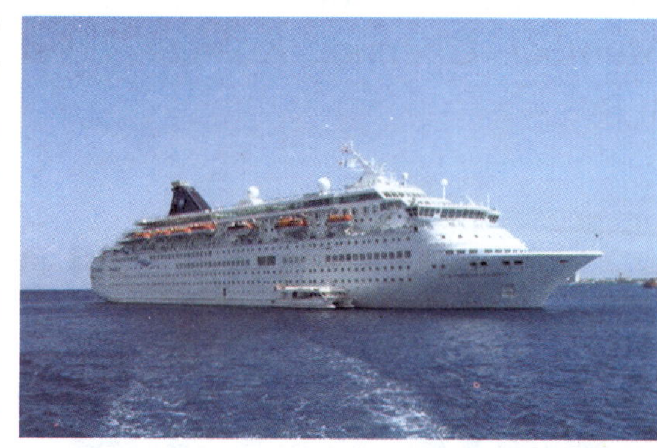

A Ship

The waterways consist of small *boats, ferries* and *steamers* moving on water bodies like *lakes* and *rivers* as well as big *watercrafts* like *ships* and *cruises* moving in seas and oceans.

Like airways, the waterways also carry passengers as well as freight together. Big watercrafts like cruises and steamers carry tonnes of freight along with a large number of passengers. Some ships are used exclusively for trading purposes and they carry only goods. Small watercrafts like boats and motorboats as well as ferries are mainly used for passenger transportation. *Canoes and rafts* are mostly used in water sports than for the purpose of transportation.

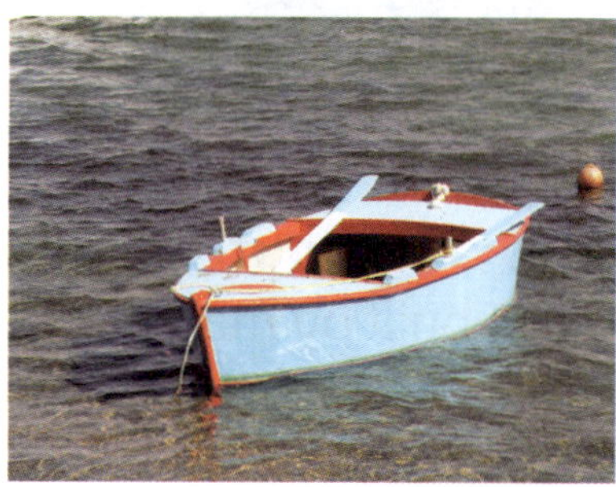

A Motor Boat

## Do You Know?

A ferry is a medium sized ship which can carry people, cargo as well as small to medium sized vehicles from one shore to another.

## Ports and Harbours

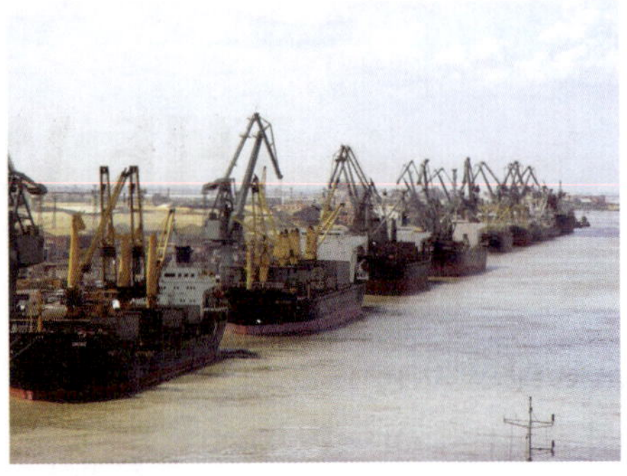

A port is a place where big trading ships are loaded and unloaded and people can embark and disembark the ships. *India has a coastline of about 7600 km.* There are as many as *13 major seaports* along the coastline. *Mumbai, Chennai, Kolkata, Paradip,*

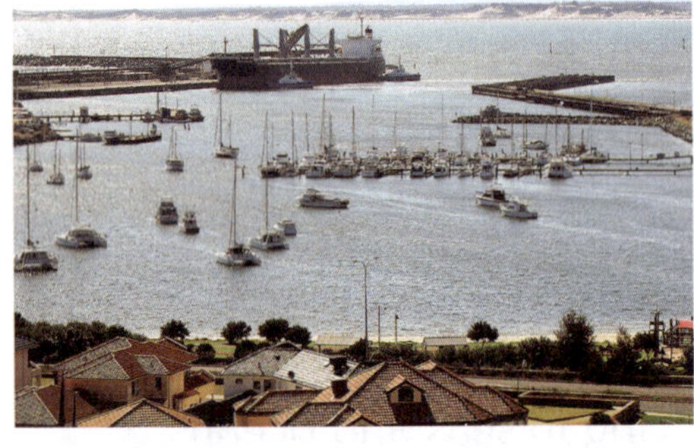

*Cochin and Port Blair* are some of the major ports. Calicut, Porbandar and Trivandrum are some of the minor ports in India.

*A harbour is a place where ships, boats and ferries take shelter.*

There are two types of harbours:

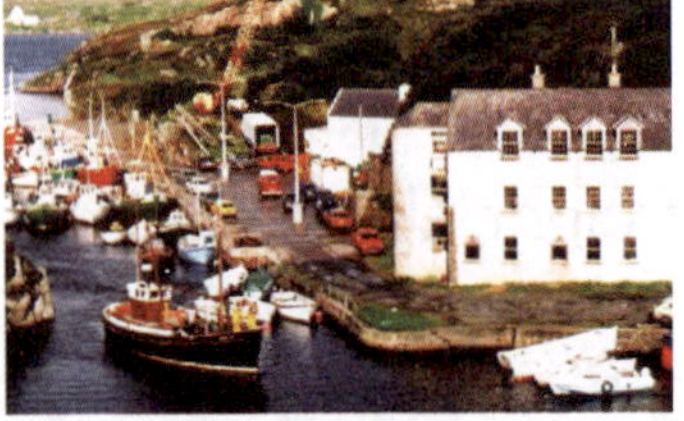

- **Natural Harbour** – It is a landform with natural cavity along the shore, where a part of the river/ sea/ ocean is protected.

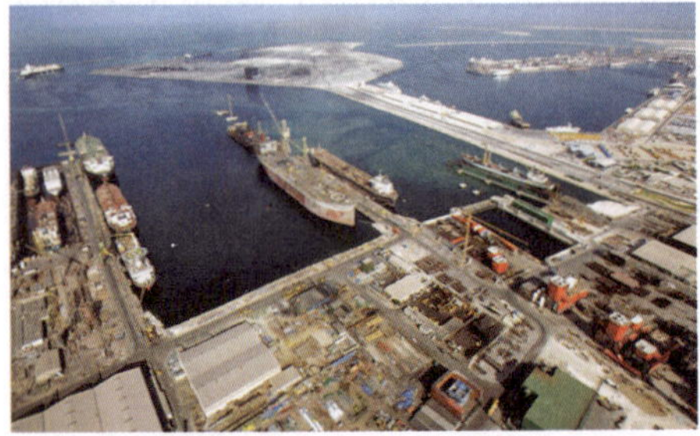

- **Artificial Harbour** – An artificial harbour is built by man along the busy sea shores to act as ports.

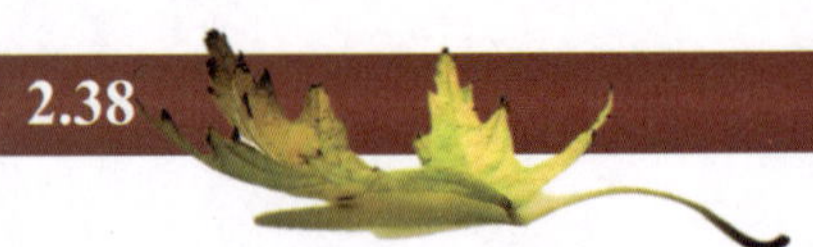

## Do You Know?

*Jebel Ali in Dubai* is the largest artificially created harbour in the world.

*Goa, Kochi, Panjim, Pondicherry and Mangalore* are some of the well-known harbours in India.

## Quick Facts

- **A peninsula is a piece of land which is surrounded by water from three sides. India is a peninsula as it is surrounded by the Bay of Bengal in the right, the Arabian Sea in the left and the Indian Ocean from below.**
- **India has an extensive network of inland waterways in the form of rivers, canals, backwaters and creeks.**
- **Ship transport is the watercraft carrying people (passengers) or goods (cargo). Sea transport has been the largest carrier of freight throughout the recorded history.**
- **The historical development of water-based transportation is connected to the importance of domestic and international trade in the world.**
- **Modern ferries, cruise ships and many types of recreational boats carry passengers for purposes ranging from daily business commuting to fishing to sightseeing. The ferry system in Halifax, Nova Scotia (Canada) demonstrates the importance of waterways for transportation.**

Chapter - 11

# SUPERSONIC MEANS OF TRANSPORTATION

A supersonic means of transportation is a vehicle which runs at a speed greater than that of the sound. In the whole universe, **sound** and **light** are the two fastest travelling entities. By developing a supersonic vehicle, man has mastered at least, one entity of this nature.

## A Supersonic Vehicle

The speed of sound is about 343.2 metres/second or 768 miles/hour. A supersonic vehicle has a faster speed than that.

The idea of an automobile with a speed greater than that of sound started fascinating scientists and researchers in the early 1950s. Since then, scientific technology has been able to develop supersonic aircraft, such as the *Concorde* and *Tupolev Tu – 144*.

## Concorde

Concorde is a supersonic aircraft used for transporting passengers. It is a product of United Kingdom.

Since their inception, a total of 20 Concordes were built by the Ministry of Civil Aviation. Out of these, around nine were purchased by state-owned airlines of Britain and France, the British Airways and the Air France.

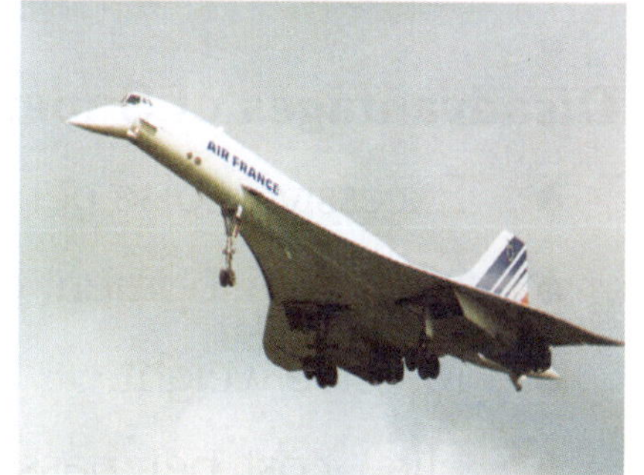

*Concorde*

## Tupolev Tu – 144

*Tupolev Tu – 144* is a Soviet supersonic aircraft. It is designed by the Soviet Tupolev Design Bureau, under the leadership of *Alexei Tupolev*.

In December 1968, Tupolev became the first supersonic plane to take flight, two months earlier than Concorde. But it was launched as a commercial air passenger after almost two years of Concorde's launch, in 1977.

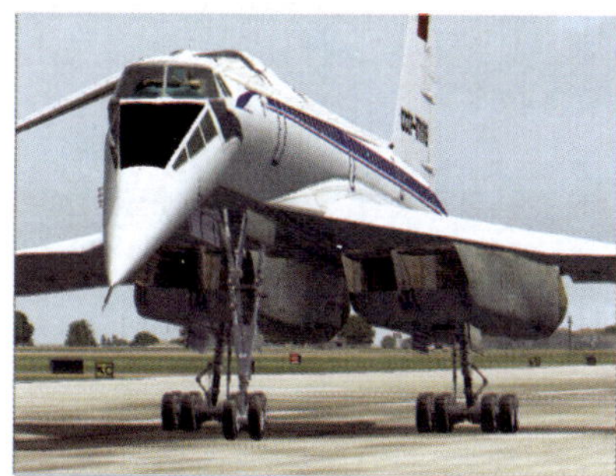

*Tupolev Tu-144*

Tupolev flew *55 scheduled passenger flights* and a total of about *102 commercial flights*. It was later used by the *National Aeronautics and Space Administration (NASA)* for supersonic research and by the Soviet Space programme to train spacecraft pilots.

## Do You Know?

The first Tupolev was unveiled in January, 1962.

### Advantages of Supersonic Transportation

- Very high speed as compared to the conventional transportation modes.
- Good efficiency, i.e., able to be more frequent, almost three times the conventional airplanes.

## Disadvantages of Supersonic Transportation

- Excessive noise generations known as *sonic booms*.
- High development cost.
- Massive weight.
- High cost per passenger as compared to the conventional airplanes.

### Quick Facts

- **Supersonic airliners' greater speed and efficiency over their conventional counterparts have made them objects of numerous recent and ongoing design studies.**
- **The drawbacks and design challenges are excessive noise generation (at takeoff and due to sonic booms during flight), high development costs, expensive construction materials, great weight, and an increased cost per seat over subsonic airliners. Despite these challenges, the Concorde was operated profitably in a niche market for over 27 years.**
- **Supersonic vehicle speeds demand narrower wing and fuselage designs, and are subject to greater stresses and temperatures. This leads to aeroelasticity problems, which require heavier structures to minimise unwanted flexing.**

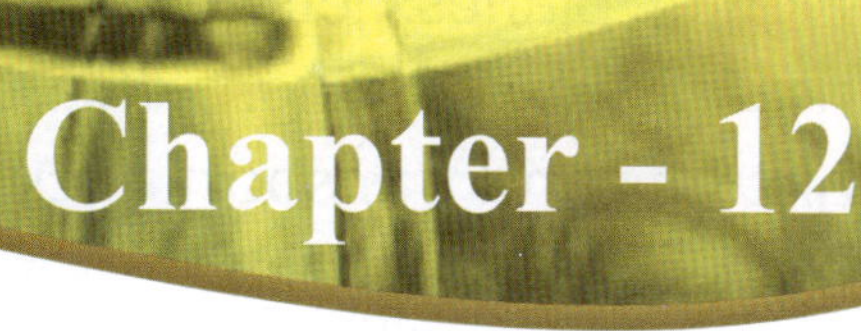

# Chapter - 12

# TRANSPORTATION IN ARMED FORCES

Armed Forces are a very important part of a nation. *Transportation plays a significant role in the defence of a country.*

**Transportation through Roadways –** Roads play an important role in defence. Roadways allow tanks and artilleries to be smoothly transported to the front.

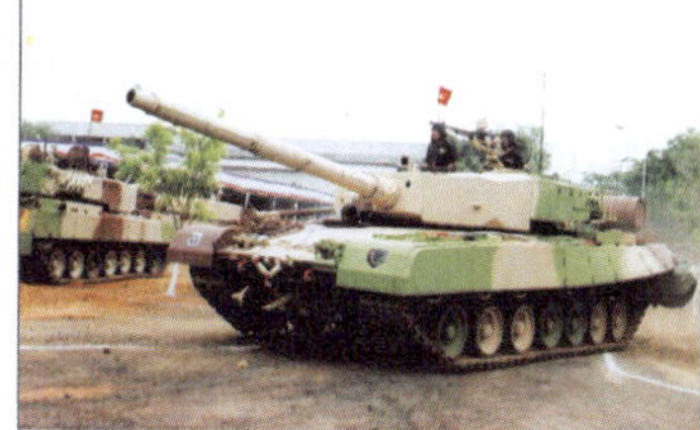

## Uses:

- Ease of transportation of soldiers, tanks, missiles and weapons to the front.
- Helps in carrying rations and other requirements to the army camps.
- Tanks equipped with radars help in locating the enemy camps.

## Do You Know?

Armed Forces are one of the firsts to help in the rescue operations in case of a disaster like earthquake, flood, tsunami.



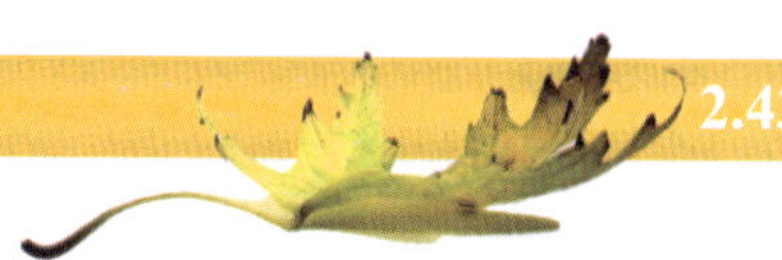

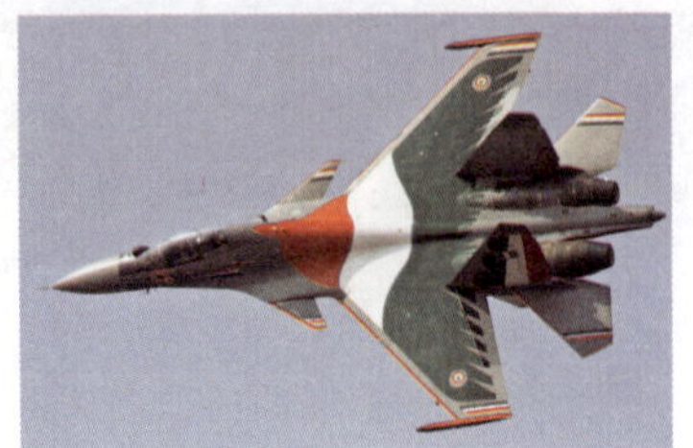

**Transportation through Airways** – Fighter planes, jets and defence helicopters use airways to fight the enemies. Tanker aircrafts and transport aircrafts are helpful in operational activities.

## Uses:

- Helps in transportation of soldiers to difficult terrains like hills and snow-capped mountains.
- Carry rations for the soldiers in difficult terrains.
- Helps in rescue operations.
- Helps in restoration work in the event of a natural calamity.

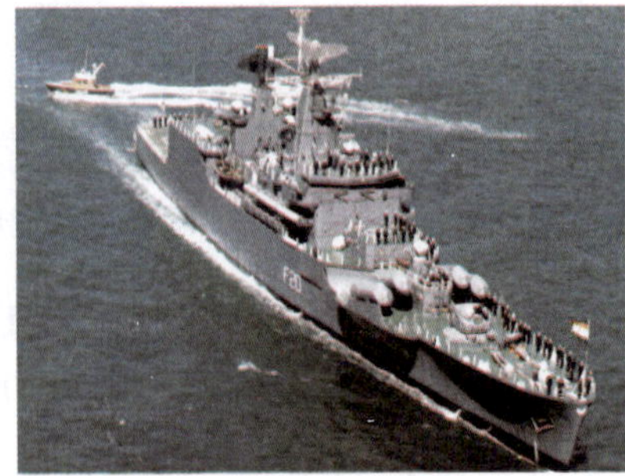

**Transportation through Waterways**– Defence services use submarines, ships, motorboats for safeguarding of the country.

## Uses:

- The Coast Guard uses ships to guard the coast of the country against smugglers, pirates and other enemies.
- The Navy uses watercrafts to defend and patrol the seas and oceans of its territory.
- Submarines gather information regarding the enemies for safe-guarding of the nation.

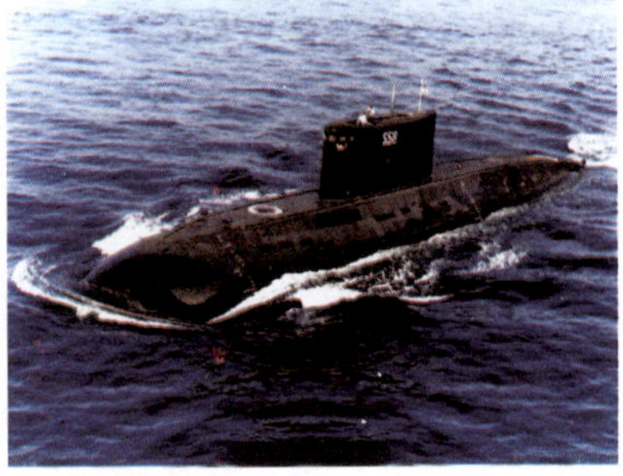

## Quick Facts

- A submarine is a water craft which moves below the surface of water (under the seas and oceans) and gathers information. The main purpose of a submarine is to be kept hidden all the time, while it collects important data and locates any danger.
- The Indian Air Force has many aircrafts of Russian, Israel, British, French, U.S. and Indian origin.
- The Indian Navy presently has one aircraft carrier ship in its active service.
- The MiG fighter planes of Russian origin have had the most number of accidents in the recent times.

Chapter - 13

# TRANSPORTATION FOR PEOPLE WITH DISABILITIES

Unlike a few decades back, the transportation scenario for disabled people has changed considerably. Many nations in the world have initiated transportation facilities for people with physical disabilities.

## Changes in Transportation Facilities

There have been many remarkable changes in the transportation facilities initiated for the disabled people.

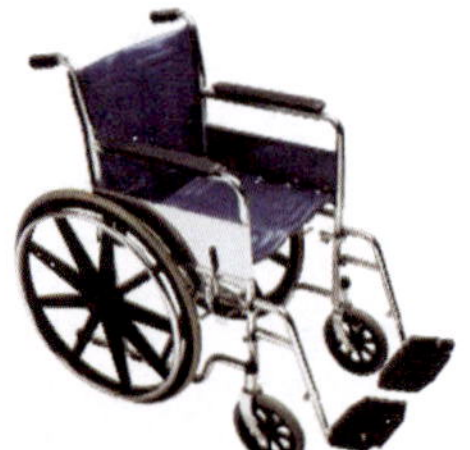

*Wheelchair*

## Private Transportation

**Wheelchair** – Automated wheelchairs with brakes are an advanced mode of transportation for physically disabled people. These are easy and efficient to use.

**Electric Scooter** – An electric scooter is the latest introduction in the domain of private

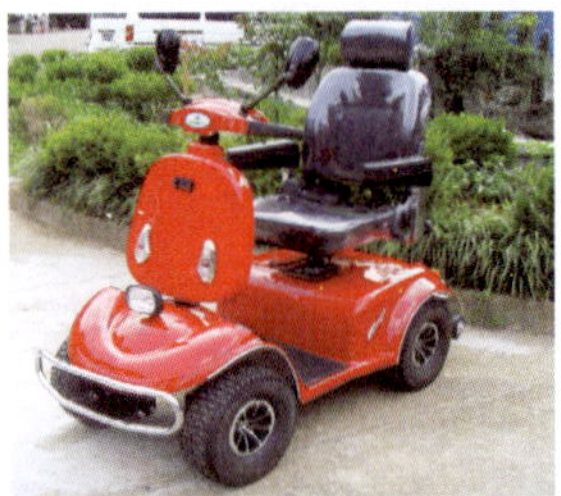

*Electric Scooter*

transportation for physically disabled people. It runs on electricity, can be recharged easily, and is compact and lightweight.

Customisation of car with low floor folding platform for easy shifting from wheelchair to car seat is readily available. Moreover, cars specially designed for disabled people are hitting the market speedily.

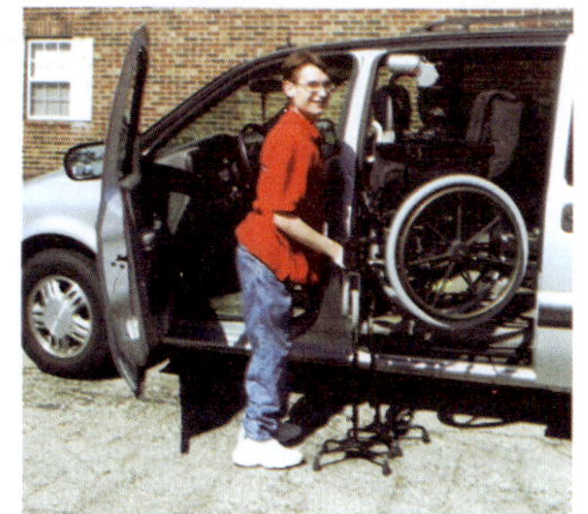

The car hand controls are available in the market. These are alternatives for car controls like brakes, clutches and accelerators, which require footwork. These hand controls are customised for people keeping in mind their handicap.

## Public Transportation

**Buses –** Low floor hybrid buses are being designed keeping in mind the disabled. They have low floors which align parallel to the bus stops and footpaths so that people on wheelchair can move into the bus without difficulty and on their own. These buses have designated space for wheelchairs, along with safety belts.

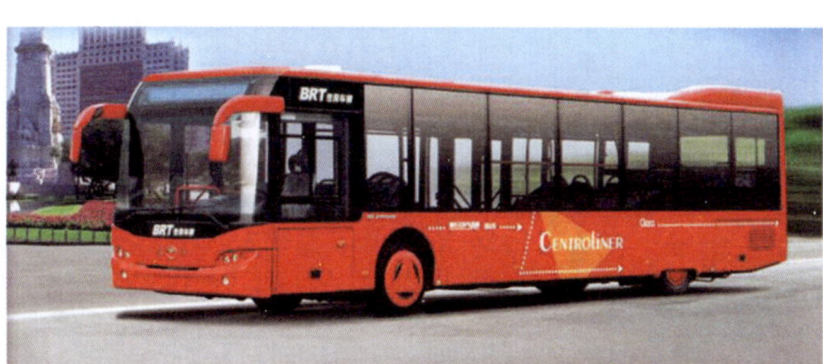


**Metro Trains –** Metro trains in Delhi is one of the most disabled-friendly public transports in the world. It provides lifts for the disabled people to move from one platform to another. Also, because the height of the platform is same to that of the metro doors, wheelchair bound people find it easy to board the train. Moreover, the space designated for disabled people makes their commuting easy and hassle-free.

**Railway Trains –** Some trains have special places reserved for wheelchairs in each compartment. This facility has not yet arrived in India. Apart from these, new constructions are being made keeping in mind the facilities for the disabled people. Footpaths are being provided with a slope for the usage of the disabled. Many public places like airports, malls, railway stations are being equipped with ramp walks.

## Quick Facts

- **The Da Paratransit Programs or ADA Paratransit Systems are run by all fixed-route bus systems in Connecticut. Each agency provides transportation for residents within their service areas who are unable to use local buses. Participants must apply for the service, provide documented proof of their disability and pay a set fee for each trip that they take, according to the Connecticut State Department of Transportation (DOT).**
- **Senior/Disabled Ride Programs: Dial-A-Ride Programs are offered by some cities or towns and community councils in Connecticut and other parts of the United States. Transportation is provided to local destinations such as banks, hospitals, stores.**
- **While technology in locomotion and mobility for the disabled has taken great strides worldwide, India is also forging ahead to modernise its age-old tricycles and wheelchairs by designing user-friendly appliances and means of transport for the disabled.**

# Chapter - 14

# TRANSPORTATION WORLDWIDE

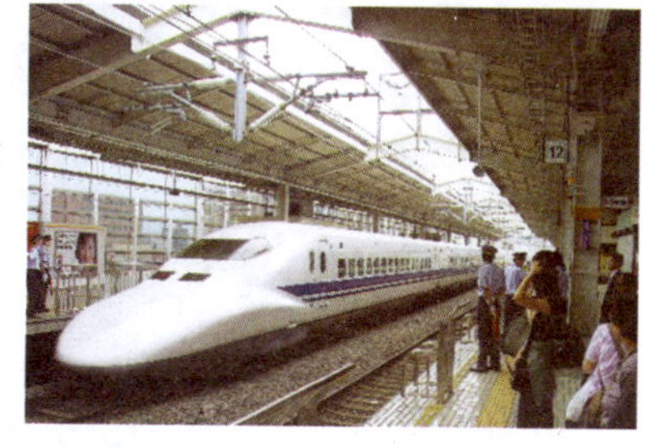

Let's have a look at the unique modes of transportation in different parts of the world. For Example, *the Bullet Train of Japan.*

Also known as *Shinkansen*, meaning 'new trunk line', the Bullet Train is one of the most famous high-speed train networks of the world. Started in 1964, this network currently has about 2,387.7 km long line. The bullet trains touch the maximum speed of 149-80 mph. A bullet can be *400m long with 16 coaches*.

According to 2007 report, around 353.18 million passengers used the bullet trains in a year.

## Aerial Tramways

*Aerial tramway*, *ropeway* or *cable car* is an aerial lift which is used for transportation mainly in the hilly regions. A cable car is a passenger cabin suspended in the air by the support of two fixed cables and propelled forward by a motor.

These cable cars are used for moving people in difficult terrains, in mining and in tourism. Recently, they have also become a part of public transport in USA – the Roosevelt Island Tramway in New York City and the Portland Aerial Tram.

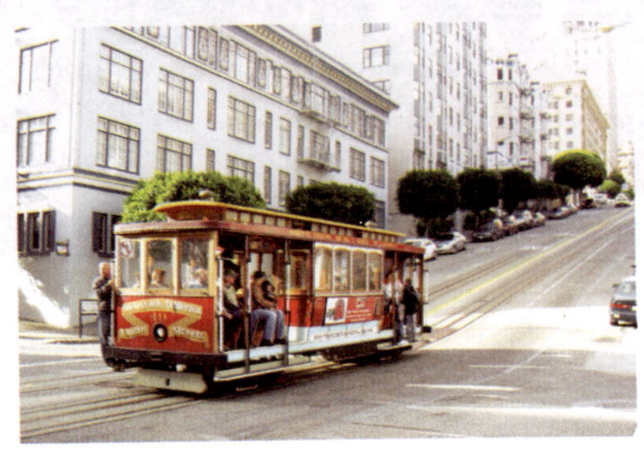

## Monorail

A monorail is a train which moves on a single rail line. The first mono rail ran in the year, 1820 in Russia. Today, there are mono rails operating in countries like South Africa, China, Japan, Singapore, Malaysia, Thailand, Philippines, Australia, America and many more.

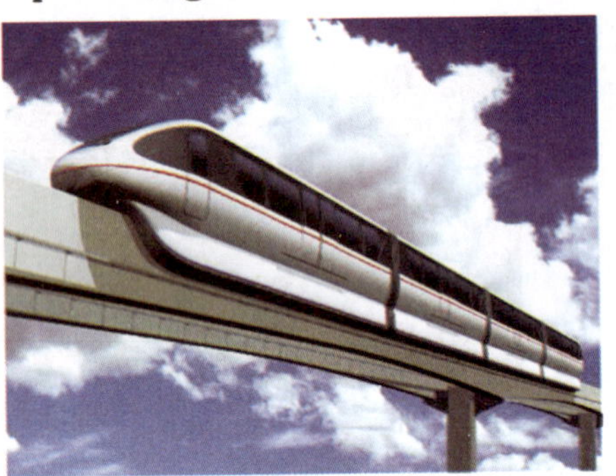

The world's busiest monorail line is the Tokyo monorail which serves approximately 127,000 passengers per day. It has served over 1.5 billion passengers since 1964.

## Trams

A tram is a passenger-carrying vehicle which runs on rail tracks laid on roads. Trams usually run within a city unlike passenger trains. They run on electricity provided by a cable running along its path. Great Britain, France, Ireland and United States have tram networks in their public transportation. The tram network in Melbourne, Australia and the Silesian Interurbans in Poland are the largest tram networks in the world. In India, Kolkata trams are the oldest in Asia, running since 1902, but now they have almost become obsolete.

## Rapid Transit

A rapid transit system is an *electric railway network* in *urban areas*. It is also known as *underground, tube, subway, or metro* in different parts of the world. The rapid transit lines are laid in the underground level of the city or on an elevated rail line in the air.

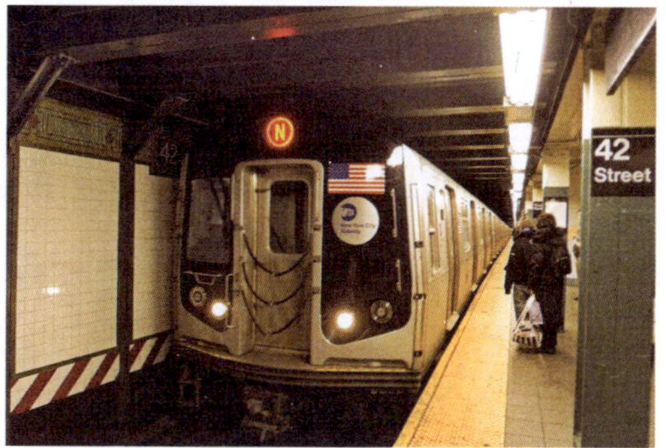


Some of the popular rapid transit networks in the world are the London Tube, the New York City Subway, the Moscow Metro, the Tokyo Subway and the Seoul Metropolitan Subway. *In India, the Kolkata Metro* was the first rapid transit network, followed by *Delhi* and *Bangalore (Bengaluru)*.

### Quick Facts

- **USA is followed up by Japan, while UK, Germany and France occupy the 3rd, 4th and 5th positions in the frequency of air travel in the world.**
- **Shipping carries most of the world's bulky goods. The desire for speedy travel has been satisfied by high-tech vessels like hydrofoils and hovercraft. Japan has around 8462 vessels followed up by Panama with 6143 vessels. USA and Russia are in the 3rd and 4th positions with 5642 and 4694 vessels respectively. China is in the 5th place.**

Chapter - 15

# FUTURISTIC MEANS OF TRANSPORTATION

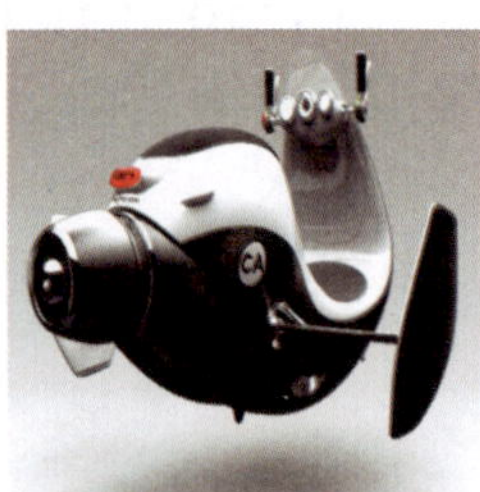
Jet Scooter

With huge daily consumption of non-renewable sources of energy for transportation, the ecological balance is getting disturbed day by day. To restore this ecological balance, we must think of some alternative sources of fuel energy to run our means of transport.

*A Jet Scooter by Norio Fujikawa of Japan* is a concept vehicle that comprises both the look of a traditional scooter and at the same time, the essence of a futuristic means of transportation. As the name denotes, this vehicle comprises a jet engine and houses only one rider.

## Solar Energy

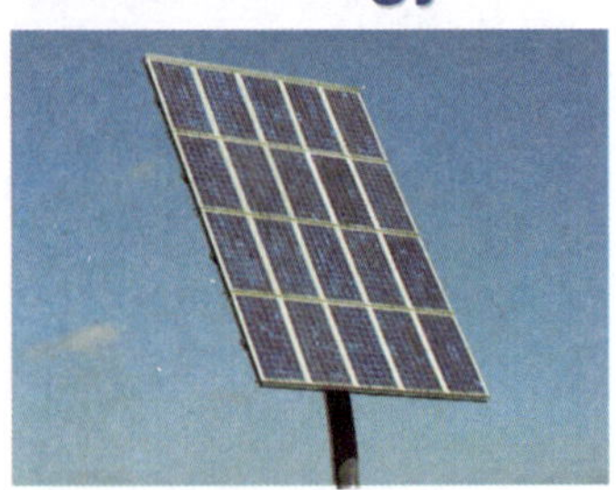
Solar Energy

Solar energy is a *never-ending source of energy*. We can make the maximum use of this source for fuelling our automobiles. The *PV cells fitted in Solar panels* can directly convert the Solar Energy into Electric Energy.

This energy can be used to run the car engine. Also, in the absence of sunlight, these solar powered vehicles can store energy and run on the backup.

Some examples of solar powered vehicles are:

**Solar Cars** – **Reva**, a solar powered car made by an Indian company can travel upto 8 km in a day.

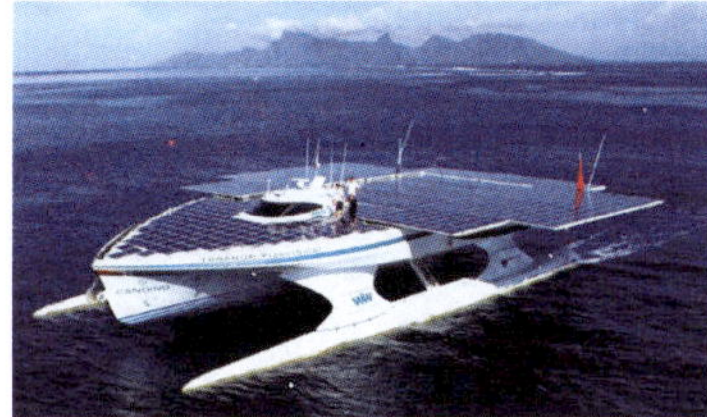

**Solar Ships** – The Turanor Planet Solar, a 30m long and 15.2m wide yacht is the world's biggest *solar powered boat*. It has an area of about 470 sq.m. of the solar panel.

**Solar Aircraft** – A lightweight solar-powered plane named *Qinetiq Zephyr*, flew in the Arizonian sky for over 336 hours. It was developed by the United Kingdom.

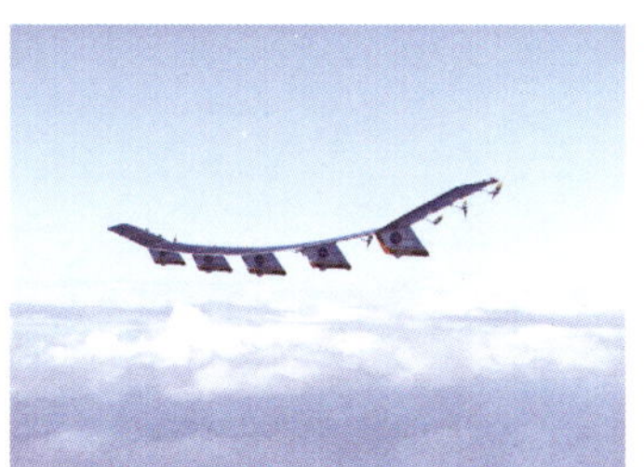

## Electricity

Electric powered vehicles are of *three types*:

- Directly powered from external power stations
- Powered by stored electricity
- Powered by an on-board electrical generator

Electric powered vehicles use direct electricity to generate power in their engines. Major car makers like *Ford Motors*, *Toyota Motors*, *Mitsubishi* are developing new generation electric vehicles. *Nissan* has manufactured their 100 percent electric car named the *Nissan Leaf*.

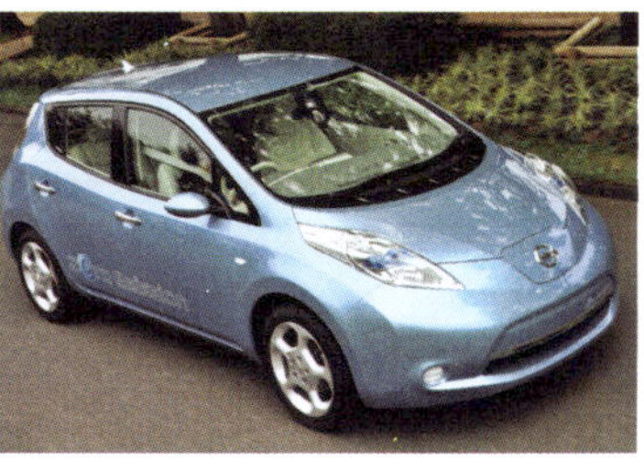

Although many public means of transport across the world like *trams* and *rapid transit systems* use electricity, but the main aim is to bring private transportation under this wing. There are millions of private automobiles running on fuels like petrol and diesel across the world. If even 50 percent of these are replaced by solar powered or electric powered vehicles, the *ecological balance* could be sustained.

## Quick Facts

- **Non-renewable sources of energy are those substances which cannot be produced in a short period of time. For example, coal, petrol and diesel are non-renewable sources as they take millions of years to form.**
- **Designed by 21-year-old Yuhan Zhang, the Volkswagen Aqua is an all-terrain hovercraft. It has an imminent approach of futuristic means of transportation powered by hydrogen and driven by impeller. Moreover, it can easily maneuver on lakes, rivers and coastal waters, to the roads, wetlands and snow and ice, with four little electric motorized fans that provide lift and thrust along with a hydrogen cell powered engine.**

# PART - II

# ELECTRONICS & COMMUNICATIONS

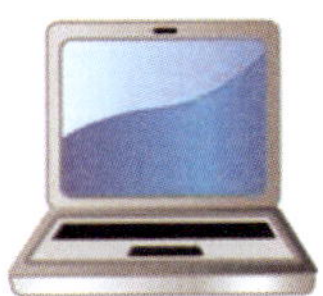
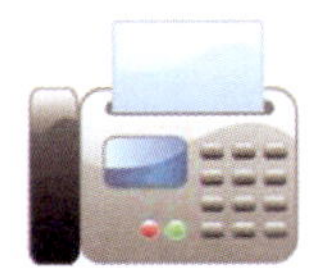
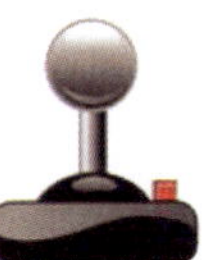
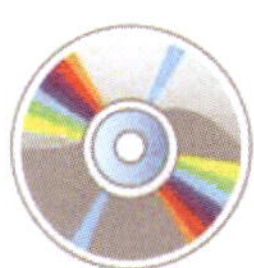
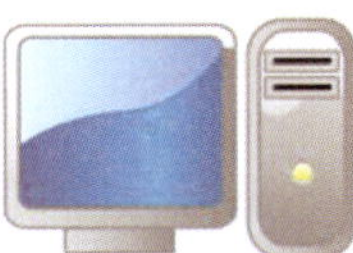
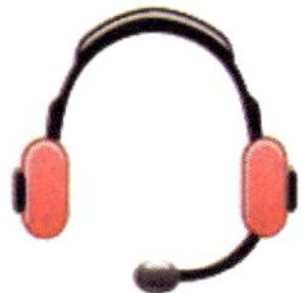
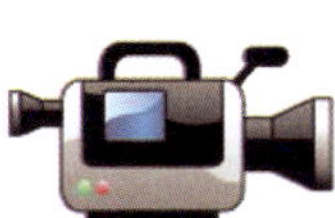
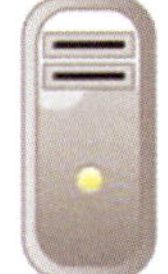
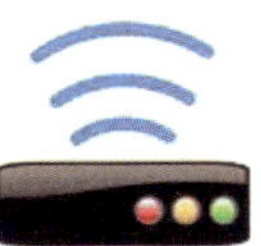

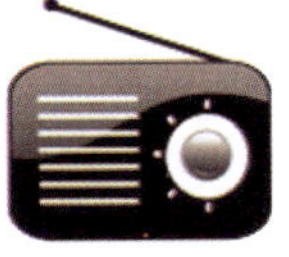
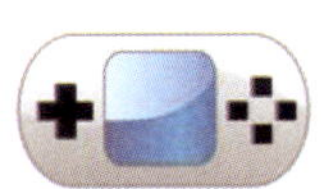
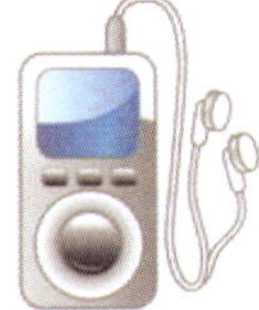
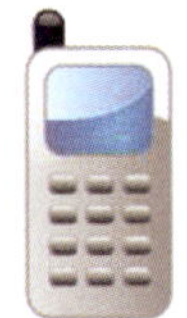
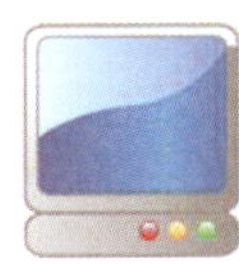
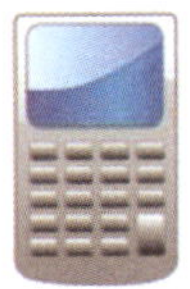
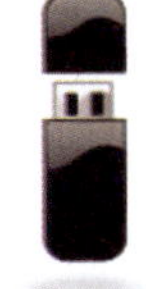
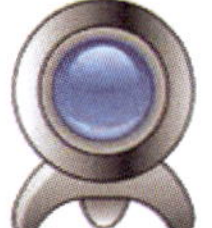
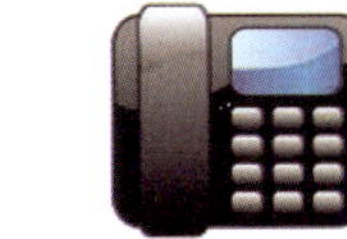
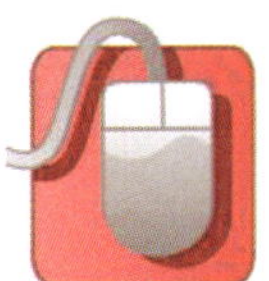
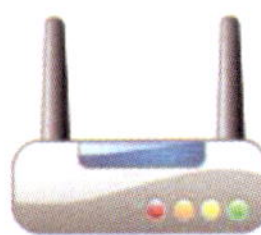
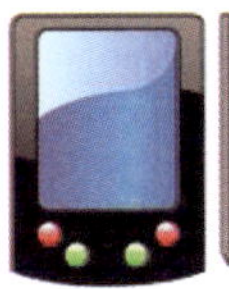
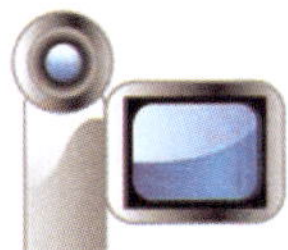
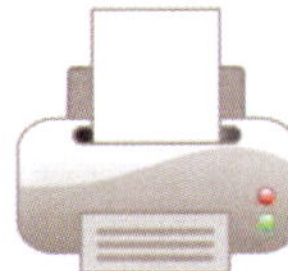
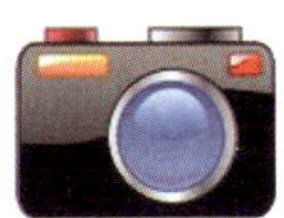

# INTRODUCTION TO ELECTRONICS

## What is Electronics?

*Electronics is a branch of Physics* which helps us in understanding various electronic devices.

**Dictionary definition –** *The science and technology of electric phenomenon is called electronics.* Under electronics, we learn various electric as well as electronic devices.

## Difference between Electrical and Electronic Devices

**Electrical –** This term relates to devices which run on electricity and are used in our day-to-day lives. For example, toaster, hair dryer, heater, radio, television.

**Electronic –** This term relates to devices which help in the construction of electrical devices. Resistors, capacitors, amplifiers and transistors are electronic devices which are used in electronic circuits of gadgets like heater, radio.

### What Constitutes Electronics?

The study of electronics covers electronic components like capacitors, resistors, inductors, diodes, transistors and different types of circuits.

An electronic component is a physical entity or an object which is used in an electric circuit. These electric circuits are used in electronic devices like radios, calculators, heaters, electric iron.

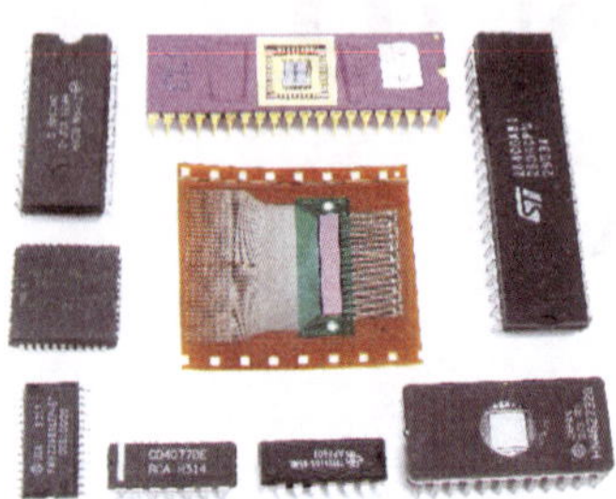

An electric circuit is a network of electronic components which are connected to each other keeping in mind various principles, laws and theories of electricity.

## Uses of Electronic Components

- These are used in the manufacturing of simple gadgets like basic radio, calculator, hand held video game.
- These are used in making electrical equipments like television, refrigerator, computer, etc.

In the following chapters, we will be learning about electronic devices like

- Transistor
- Transformer
- Capacitor
- Amplifier
- Resistor

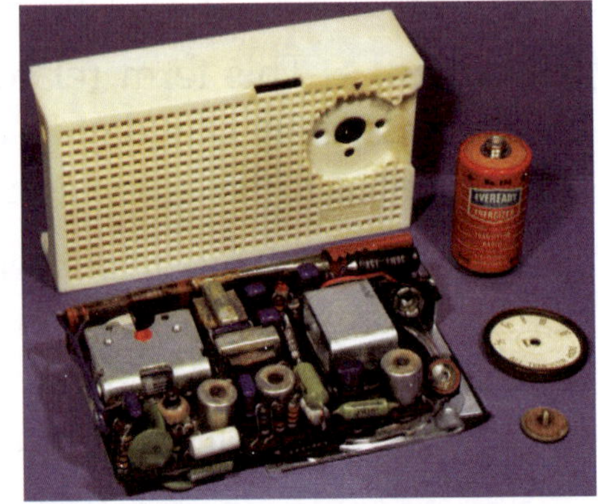

## Quick Facts

**Some exciting inventions in electronics:**

- **1600 – William Gilbert coined the term, 'electricity'.**
- **1733 – Benjamin Franklin named the two types of charges as 'positive' and 'negative'.**
- **1800 – Alessandro Volta invented an electric battery.**
- **1821 – Michael Faraday invented an electric motor.**
- **1883 – Electric transformer was invented.**
- **1907 - Lee De Forest invented the electric amplifier.**
- **1947 – Transistor was invented.**

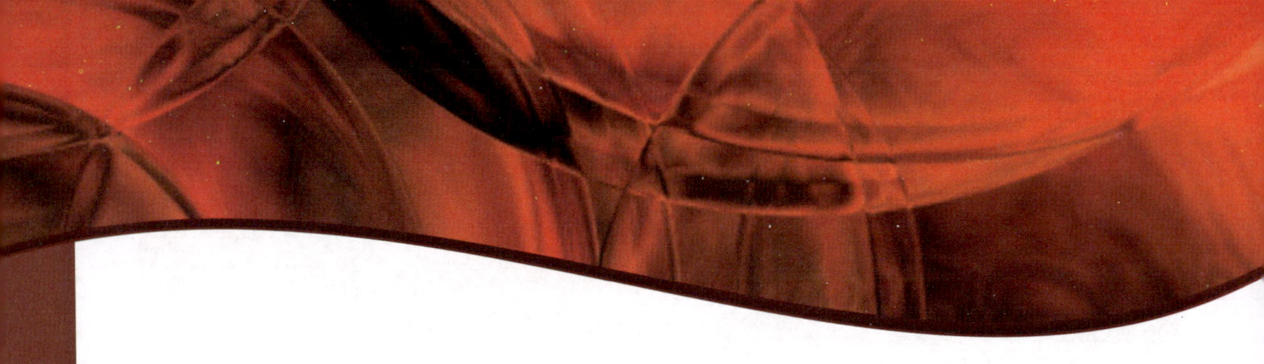

# ELECTRIC CHARGE AND ELECTRIC CURRENT

## Electric Charge

Electric charge is a *physical property of matter*. When matter comes in contact with a charged particle, it experiences a force. This is because it goes through an attraction or repulsion between the electric charge present inside it and the charge it comes in contact with.

## Electric Charge is of Two Types:

- Positive charge
- Negative charge

| Positive Charge | Negative Charge | Result |
|---|---|---|
| + | - | Attraction |
| + | + | Repulsion |
| - | - | Repulsion |
| - | + | Attraction |

When two opposite charges come in contact with each other, they experience **attraction**. This is called an *attractive charge*.

For example, a positively charged matter coming in contact with a negatively charged matter experiences an attractive force.

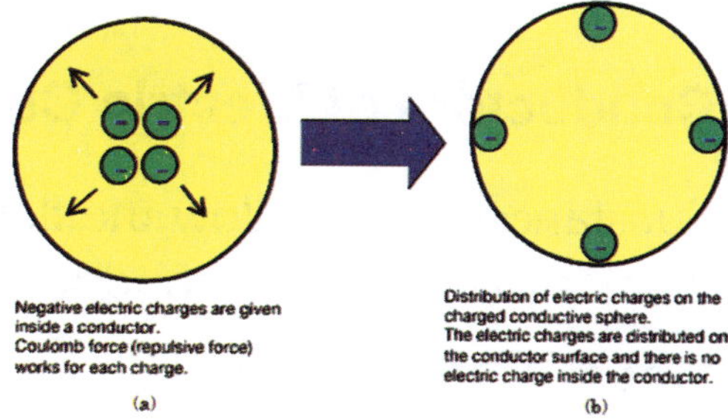
Negative electric charges are given inside a conductor. Coulomb force (repulsive force) works for each charge.
(a)
Distribution of electric charges on the charged conductive sphere. The electric charges are distributed on the conductor surface and there is no electric charge inside the conductor.
(b)

When two similar charges come in contact with each other, they experience **repulsion**. This is called a *repulsive charge*.

For example, positively charged matter coming in contact with another positively charged matter experiences a repulsive force.

## Unit of Electric Charge

The SI unit of an electric charge is **coulomb**. It is denoted by a capital **'C'**.

## Electric Current

*Flow of electric charge through a medium is called electric current.* An electric current is generated when *electrons move through a conductor like wire*. It is very similar to water flowing through a pipe.

When electrons continuously move through a conductor such as wire, electric current is generated. This electric current, or simply called current, is used to run various electronic devices like tube light, fan, motor, microwave, refrigerator.

## Unit

The SI unit of electric current is **ampere**. It is denoted by a capital **'A'**.

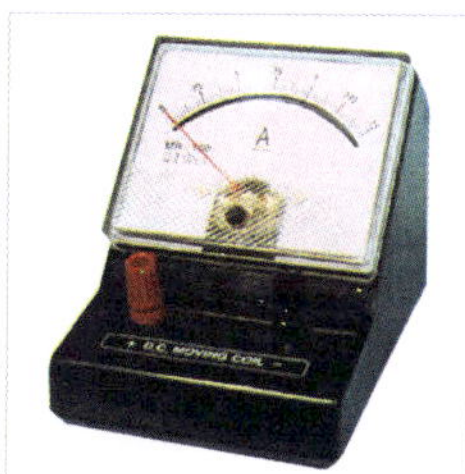

Ampere = 1 coulomb per second

The amount of electric current is measured using an **ammeter**.

## Conductors of Electric Current

Substances which allow the flow of electric charge (or electrons) in themselves are called conductors of electric current.

**Good Conductors –** Most metals like copper, aluminium, iron are good conductors of electricity. Graphite being a non-metal is also a good conductor of electric current.

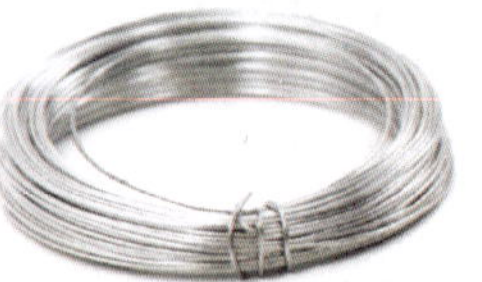

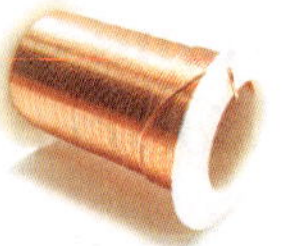

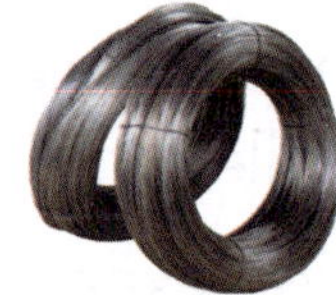

**Bad Conductors –** Most non-metals like wood, glass, rubber are bad conductors of electric current.

*Electric energy is easily transportable via integrated electric grids.* After transportation, electric energy is converted into mechanical energy, thermal energy, light energy, and chemical energy.

### Quick Facts

- **When an electric charge builds up on the surface of an object, it creates static electricity.**
- **Electricity is by no means a purely human invention, and may be observed in several forms in nature, such as lightning.**
- **A generator is a device that converts mechanical energy into electrical energy. The process is based on the relationship between magnetism and electricity.**

- Electric eels can produce strong electric shocks of around 500 volts for both self defence and hunting.
- Electric energy is an intermediate form of energy. It is produced in thermal power stations (where fuel oil, gas, coal, biomass are burnt), in hydroelectric power stations and nuclear power stations. Smaller quantities are produced by wind, photovoltaic solar panels, sea tides.
- Demand for solar electric energy has consistently grown by 20-25% per year over the past 20 years.
- In 1791, Luigi Galvani published his discovery of bioelectricity, demonstrating that electricity was the medium by which nerve cells passed signals to the muscles.
- In 1882, water was used to electrify two paper mills and a house on the Fox River. The Fox River is a tributary of the Illinois River in the United States. This was the first application of hydroelectric energy.

# Chapter - 3

# TRANSISTOR

Transistor is a very basic and essential device in most of the electronic devices. A transistor is a semiconductor device which is used to *amplify* and *switch electronic signals*.

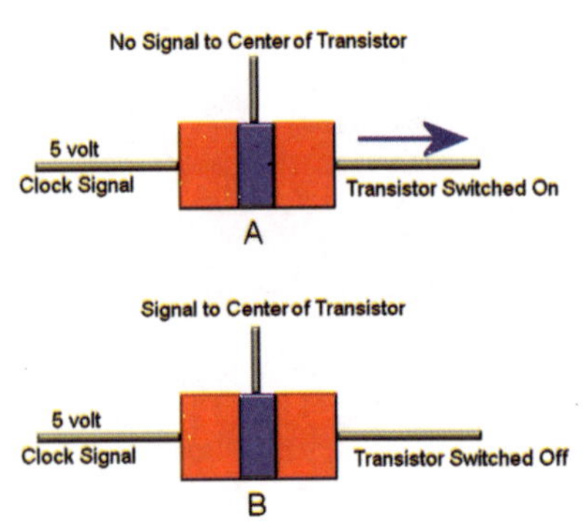


## Working of a Transistor

Transistors have two main functions – *amplifying* and *switching*.

## Transistor as an Amplifier

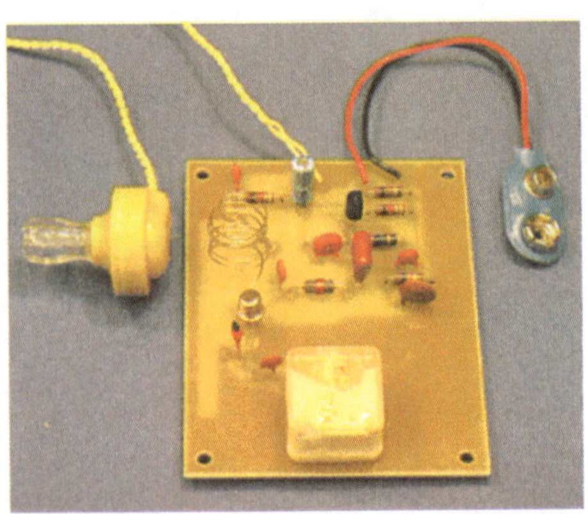

A transistor works as a gatekeeper for current in an electronic device. It is made up of three parts – a base, a collector and an emitter. The collector is like an inlet of the current flow to the base. The base acts as a gate to the flow of electric current. It regulates the current and sends the regulated current to the emitter.

This whole process is similar to using a tap to control the flow of water supplied from the main pipes.

## Transistor as a Switch

A transistor works in the same way as an amplifier by regulating the flow of current. After regulating the amount, it makes sure that a specific amount of electric current goes out through the emitter. If the amount of current is equal to the specified amount, the transistor 'switches-on'. If the amount of current is less than the specified amount, the transistor 'switches-off'.

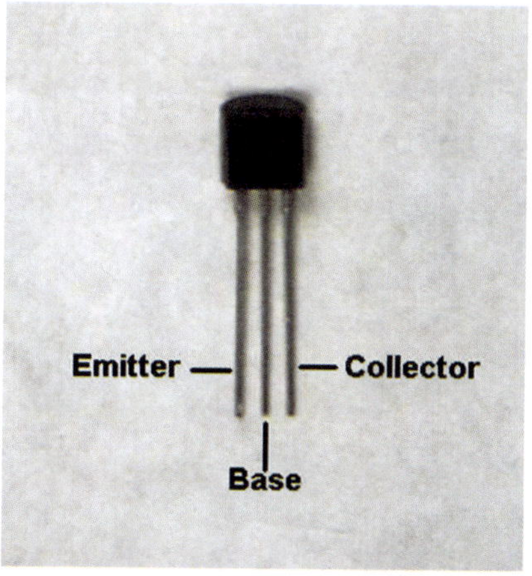


## Do You Know?

John Bardeen, Walter Brattain and William Shockley are the scientists who invented the transistor in the year, 1947.

### Advantages of Using a Transistor

A transistor is a fundamental unit of modern electronic devices. Devices like radio, calculators, computers, telephones use transistors.

**Mass Produced –** Good quality transistors can be produced in large quantities.

**Low Cost –** Because of their mass production, transistors are very inexpensive.

**Flexibility –** Transistors are preferred for writing computer programs than to design complex functions in computers.

## Quick Facts

- Semiconductor – A semiconductor is a substance which allows the flow of electric current under specific conditions. Thus, it is useful in regulating the electric current.
- Amplify – The term, 'amplify' means to increase strength.
- The first commercial device to use the transistor was the Sonotone 1010 hearing aid.
- Early transistors were used to amplify audio signals.
- The first transistor radio went on the market in 1954 and had only four transistors.
- Gordon Moore, co-founder of Intel, predicted that the number of transistors on a chip would double about every two years. This is known as Moore's Law.

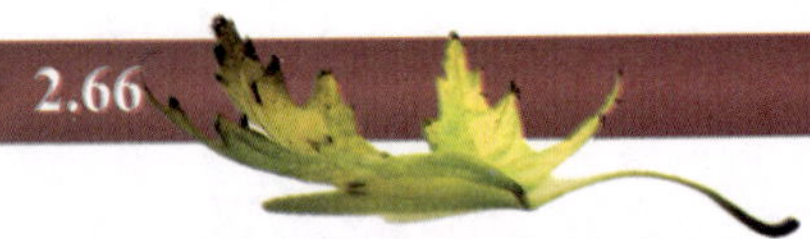

Chapter - 4

# TRANSFORMER

A transformer is an electronic device which is used to *transfer electric current from one circuit to another*.

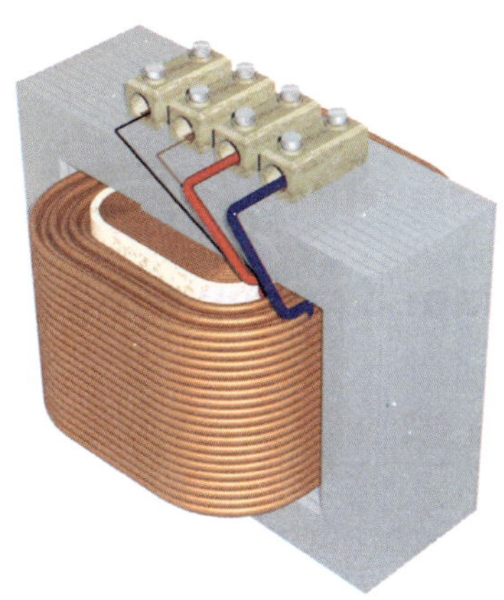

## Electric Current

The electricity you get in your house comes to you through a big transformer. The electricity board transmits electric current through wires to a transformer in your residential area. This transformer then distributes the electricity to each and every house of the area. If there was no transformer, the electric current coming straight from electricity board to your house would be very high and would destroy the electric circuit in your house. Then you won't be able to run a tube light or a fan.

## Construction of a Transformer

A transformer is a device made up of an *insulated metal core* (usually iron). The two parallel arms of the iron core are coiled with copper wires. These two coils are called primary and secondary winding.

## Working of a Transformer

Primary winding of the transformer gets the input voltage which is converted from low voltage to high voltage or vice-versa. To convert low voltage to high voltage, the coils in the secondary windings are increased. To convert high voltage to low voltage, the coils in the secondary windings are decreased.

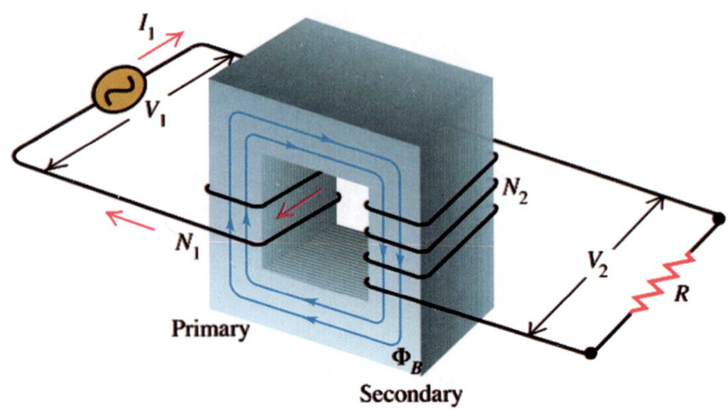


## Do You Know?

**William Stanley** designed the first transformer in the year **1885**.

## Uses of a Transformer

- Transformers modify electric current under difficult conditions like low voltage to high voltage, high voltage to low.
- They distribute electricity over long distances.
- They protect electronic devices from a huge load of electric current.
- They lower the main voltage to a usable level for an electronic device.
- They filter out any problem in the conductor.

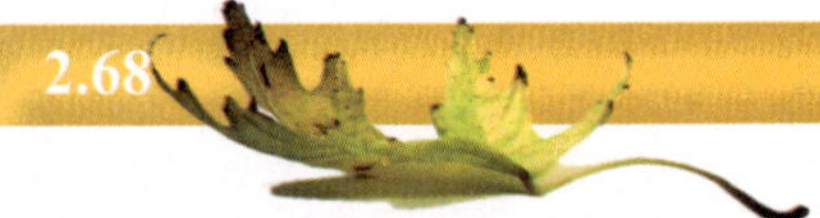

## Quick Facts

- Voltage, also known as electric tension, is the energy required to move electric current from one point to another. It is measured in 'volts' and is denoted by a capital 'V'.
- Generally, a voltage of 220V is required to run electric equipments
- A circuit is a path between the start point and the end point of the flow of electric current.
- Basically, a transformer is an electrical device used to transfer an alternating current or voltage from one electric circuit to another by the means of electromagnetic induction.

# Chapter - 5

# CAPACITOR

A capacitor is an electronic device used to store *electrical energy*.

## Construction of a Capacitor

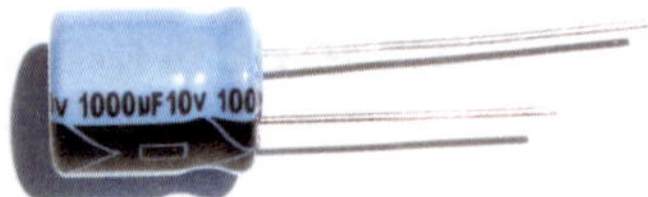


A capacitor is made up of *two conducting plates*, usually metals, at two ends and a non-conducting plate called a 'dielectric' in between them.

## Working of a Capacitor

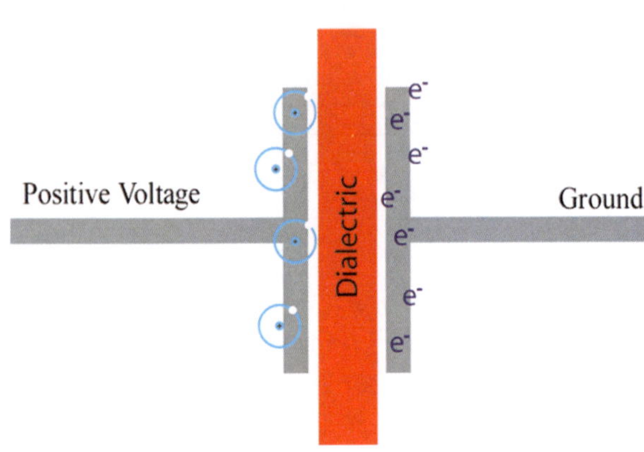


When there is a **voltage** *fluctuation* across the conductors in a capacitor, an electric field appears across the **dielectric**. This causes positive charge to collect on one conductor and negative charge on another conductor. The energy generated is thus stored in this **electric field**.

## Uses of a Capacitor

- Capacitors are widely used in electric circuits of many electrical devices.
- They are used in filter networks for the smooth flow of power supplies.
- They are used in circuits inside a radio to tune into the desired FM station.

## Making Your Own Capacitor

**Things Required –** copper wire, wire strippers, cling film, aluminium foil, cellotape and scissors.

**Procedure:**

1. Take two pieces of copper wires. Remove 2 cm of plastic covering from the copper wire using wire stripper.
2. Place a piece of cling film on the table. Make sure there isn't any wrinkle.
3. Place a piece of aluminium foil 1cm shorter than the cling film.
4. Attach the end of the stripped copper wire on the aluminium foil with the help of a cellotape. The copper wire and the aluminium foil must remain in contact with each other.
5. Now place another piece of the cling film on the aluminium foil. Repeat steps 2 to 4 again.
6. Roll the whole thing into a cylinder with the cling film on the outside.
7. Put the cellotape on the cylinder in order to hold all things together.
8. Now the aluminium foil acts as a *conductor* and the cling film as a *dielectric*.

## Quick Facts

- A dielectric is another term used for insulators/ bad conductors of electric current.
- An electric field is a virtual space surrounding the electrically charged particles.
- The concept of electric field was introduced by Michael Faraday.
- Capacitors contain a circuit, light and a switch. Because of the ability of the capacitor to block flow of the current it is often used as a filter.
- A capacitor cannot produce new electrons. It can store electrons only.
- The unit of capacitance is called a farad. A 1-farad capacitor is able to store one coulomb of charge at one volt.
- Super capacitors are electric double layer capacitors which have a capacitance of 0.47 Farad.

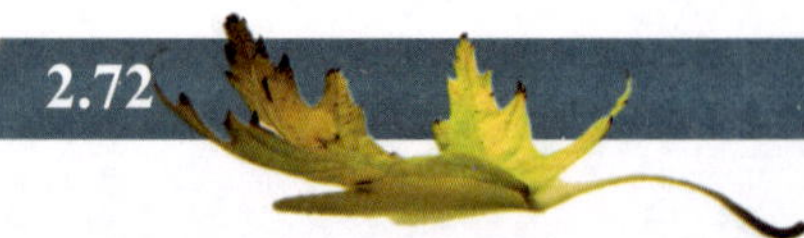

Chapter - 6

# INDUCTOR

*An inductor is a two-terminal electronic device which is used to store energy in a magnetic field.* It is also known as a **reactor** or a **coil**. It is a basic component which is used in devices where voltage and current change.

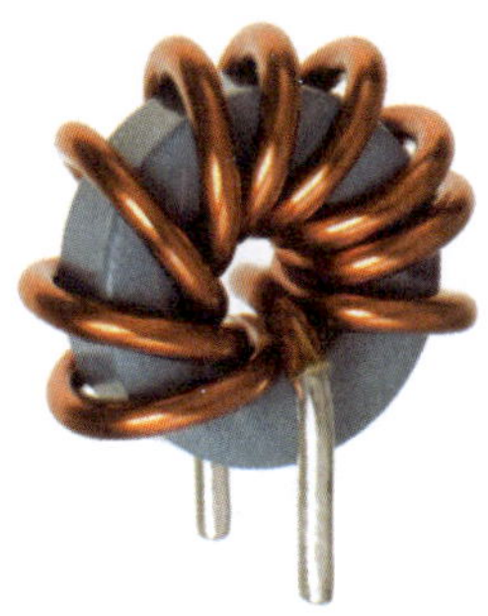

## Construction of an Inductor

An inductor is a coil of conducting material (such as copper wire) wound on a permanently magnetised iron core.

## Working of an Inductor

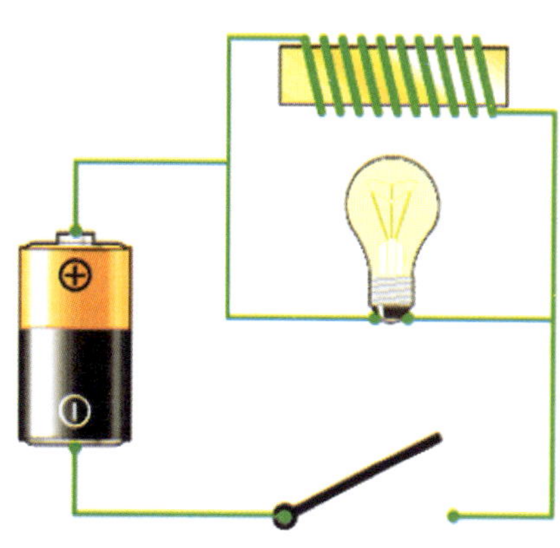

An inductor is simply a wire coil wrapped on a magnetised iron core. It opposes the flow of electric current. When a voltage is applied to a coil of wire, a magnetic field is created around the coils. This magnetic field gives birth to an opposing **voltage**. As voltage is the process of flow of electric current, therefore, the inductor opposes this current.

## Uses of an Inductor

- Large inductors are used in power supplies.
- Small inductors are used in circuits used in radio reception and transmission.
- They are used to decrease the voltage from lightning strikes.
- They are used to limit faulty currents in a device.

## Making Your Own Inductor

**Things Required**:

A copper wire, 6 inches long, a bar magnet, an iron nail

**Procedure:**

1. A bar magnet has two magnetic poles at its two ends – south and north. Decide which polarity you want to give your iron nail.
2. Place the iron nail horizontally on the table. Gently rub one end of the bar magnet from head of the nail to its tail.
3. Repeat this action continuously for 5-10 minutes with the same end of the magnet.
4. Now, start winding the copper wire on the middle of the nail tightly.
5. Your inductor is ready.

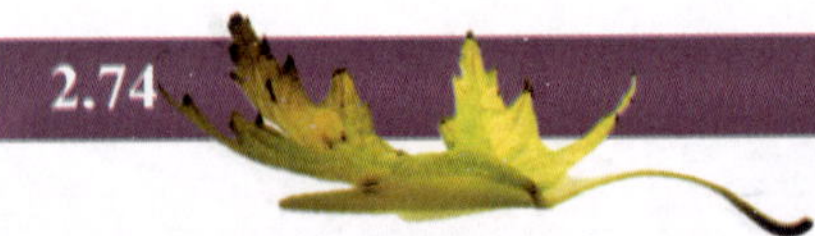

## Quick Facts

- A magnetised iron core is that which has been made permanently magnetic in nature by keeping in contact with a magnetic field for a long time.
- The inductor stores electrical energy in the form of magnetic energy.
- The inductor does not allow Alternating Current (AC) to flow through it, but does allow Direct Current (DC) to flow through it.
- Typical applications for inductors used in power supply circuits are "voltage conversion" and "choke," and these inductors are used in a wide range of electronic equipment.
- Inductors store electrical energy in magnetic fields.
- They act as open circuit at first when we apply DC (Direct Current) to them, but after a while, they freely allow it to pass.
- They oppose to changes in current.

Chapter - 7

# RESISTOR

Resistors are very common elements of electronic circuits and electrical networks. A resistor is a device which opposes the flow of electric current in a circuit. It controls and impedes the passage of current.

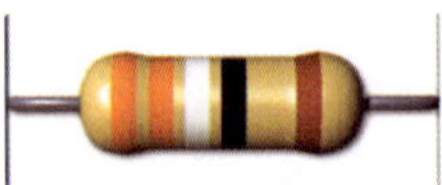

## Unit

Resistors offer resistance to a device. This property is measured in Ohm. It is symbolised as Ω.

## Construction of a Resistor

A basic resistor is made up of powdered carbon bound by an adhesive like glue. It has two metal wires at both ends of its cylindrical body.

## Do You Know?

The coloured stripes on the body of a resistor help in calculating the value of that resistor.

## Working of a Resistor

A resistor works to break the flow of current in a device. Let's



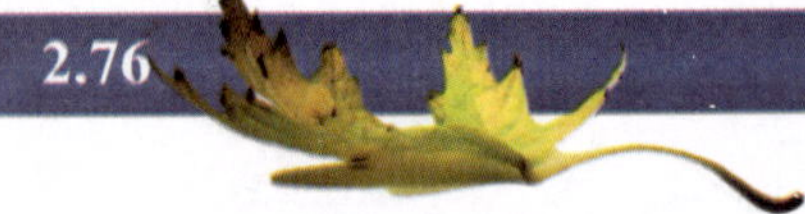

understand this with the help of an example. Imagine water flowing through a pipe. If we decrease the diameter of the mouth of the pipe, the amount of water flowing out would decrease. This is because now diameter is reduced so more resistance.

## Types of Resistors

Fixed resistors – These are resistors whose values are fixed.

Variable resistors – These are resistors whose values can be increased or decreased while connected to a circuit.

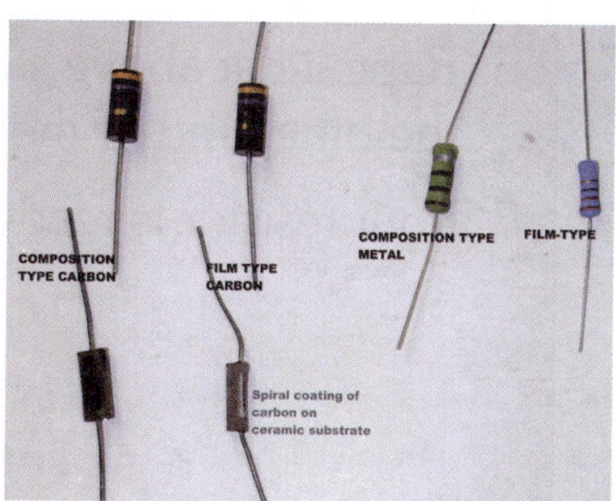


*Types of Resistors*

## Uses of a Resistor

- They are used in television and radio circuits.
- They are used as heating elements in heaters, irons, toasters.
- They are used as filaments in light bulbs.

## Making your own Resistor

Things required – A pencil, knife/cutter, two pieces of 6-inch copper wire, soldering iron, a nail (same thickness as of the pencil lead), a wooden board.

## Procedure

1. Remove the lead from the pencil with the help of a knife/cutter. Be careful while doing this.
2. Fix a nail on a wooden board.
3. Take a piece of copper wire. Tightly wind a 2 inches wire on the nail.

4. Your wire will get a spiral shape. Repeat the above step with the second wire.
5. Now insert one end of the pencil lead into the spiral part of the copper wire. Bind it with the help of solder iron.
6. Repeat the above step with the second piece of copper wire on the other end of the lead.
7. Your resistor is ready.

## Quick Facts

- **Resistors are used to create a known voltage to the current ratio in an electric circuit.**
- **The higher the value of resistance which is measured in ohms, the lower the current will be.**
- **Resistors are colour coded. Look for the colour stripe on the resistor indicating which way the current is flowing. The power flows from the end without the stripe to the end with the stripe.**
- **The Ohm's Law states that the potential difference between the two points on a resistor and the current flowing through it must be proportional. The electrical resistance is equal to the voltage drop across the resistor divided by the current through the resistor.**

# Chapter - 8

# USES OF ELECTRONICS

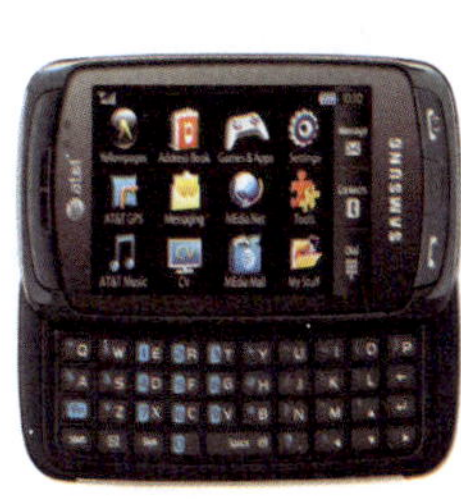

Since the beginning of modern age, the world has seen many great inventions in the field of science and technology. The advent of electricity is one of many such great inventions. The electric and electronic devices we use today are based on these inventions. These devices have become important and significant part of our life. Today, we can't imagine our lives without electric gadgets as they have become indispensable for us.

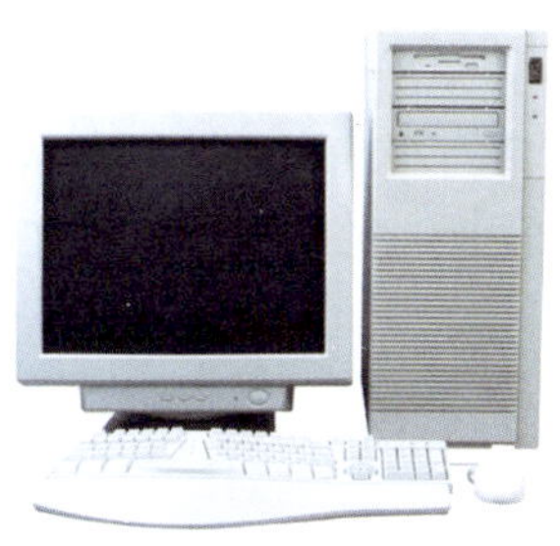

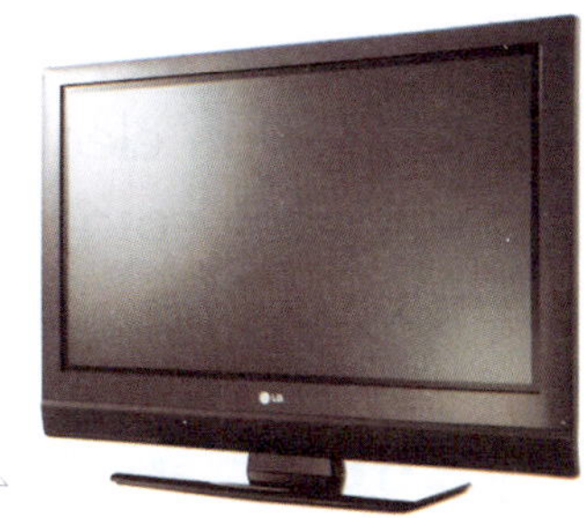

In the previous chapters, we have read about many small and basic electronic devices like *transistors, transformers, capacitors, amplifiers and resistors*. These are mere components for the production of gadgets like radio, computer, television, cell phones. But, without them, these gadgets don't have any foundation.

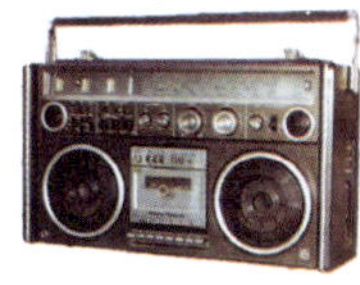

Let us learn some important and significant uses of electronic devices.

## Communication

*Electronic devices like radio, television, internet, phones* are the biggest and popular means of communication today. These devices and gadgets help us connect with the world at large.

## Medical Health Care

Electronic devices find their way in modern day medical health care through machines like *MRI, CAT, CT scan, X-ray scan*. Electronic equipments like pacemakers are a gift to humans beings.

## Transportation

Vehicles like *aeroplanes, helicopters, metro, bullets* use electric and electronic technologies. This ensures better speed and comfort at low cost, while saving the time of transportation.

## Research and Development

*Fibre optical, nano technology, wireless technology* – all these had their basis on electronic components. Development of spacecrafts, satellites and other new techniques require the help of electronic technology.

## Electronic Trading

With the advent of *internet, electronic trading* has developed at a very fast pace. People use internet for trading, and they use credit and debit cards for shopping.

## Entertainment

People use mobile phones, digital cameras, music players, laptops,

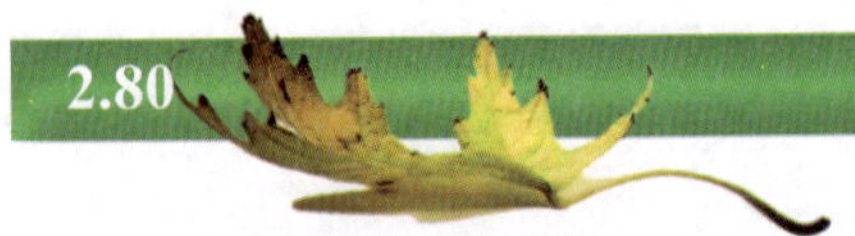

television to entertain themselves. Electronic devices have made life much more enjoyable than before.

## General Use

From a remote control to a coffee grinder, electronic devices are making their presence felt at every step of our lives. Today, they are a part of our daily routine.

### Quick Facts

- Electronics are the basis of many modern technologies, from hi-fl systems to missile control systems.
- Electronics are systems which control things by automatically switching tiny electrical circuits on and off.
- Transistors are electronic switches. They are made of materials called semiconductors that change their ability to conduct electricity.
- Diodes are transistors with two connectors. They control an electric current by switching it on or off.
- Triodes are transistors with three connectors that amplify the electric current (make it bigger) or reduce it.
- A silicon chip consists of thousands of transistors linked together by thin metal strips in an integrated circuit, on a single crystal of the semi-conductor, silicon.
- The electronic areas of a chip are those treated with traces of chemicals, such as boron and phosphorus, which alter conductivity of silicon.

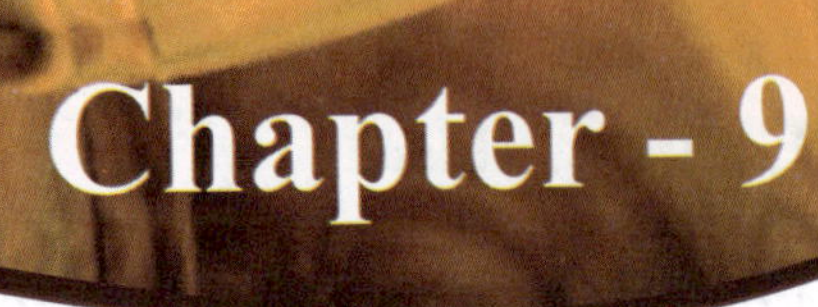


# INTRODUCTION TO COMMUNICATION

## What is Communication?

Communication is a process by which a person can deliver his message to another person.

The term, 'communication' is derived from the Latin word, *communis*, which means 'to share'.

We use communication to express our views and opinions and listen to other's views and opinions. Communication is also a process through which we send across important information and receive a feedback.

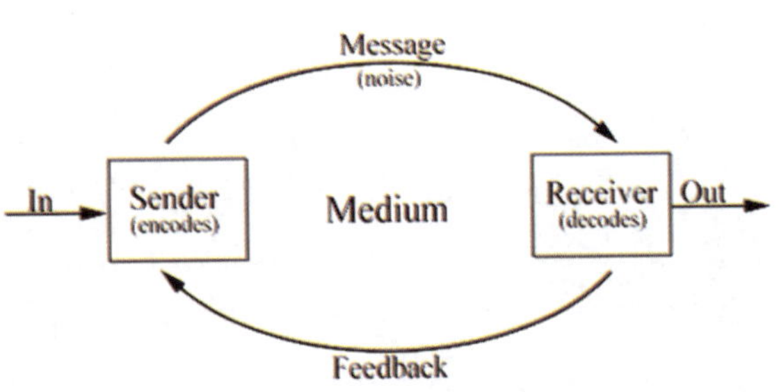


## Elements of Communication:

- **Sender –** A person or a group of persons who want to communicate or send a message

- **Message** – A piece of information which needs to be shared
- **Receiver** – A person or group of persons to whom the message is directed

We communicate through following mediums:

- Speaking
- Body language
- Writing letters
- Telephone
- Newspapers
- Radio
- Television
- Internet

## Beginning of Communication

The need to express himself/herself to others is one of the main needs of a human being, apart from air, water and food.

Since the evolution of the earth, man has tried to communicate with others through various ways. When there was no language, man tried to communicate through gestures and sounds. Later, he used pictures and drawings to communicate. Some of the pictographs found in archaeological sites of Mesopotamian and Indus Valley Civilization are perfect examples of man's efforts to express himself.

The advent of language made it easier for the early man to express himself. He could now communicate easily. The invention of grammar and scripts made it all the more easier for him to write and express.

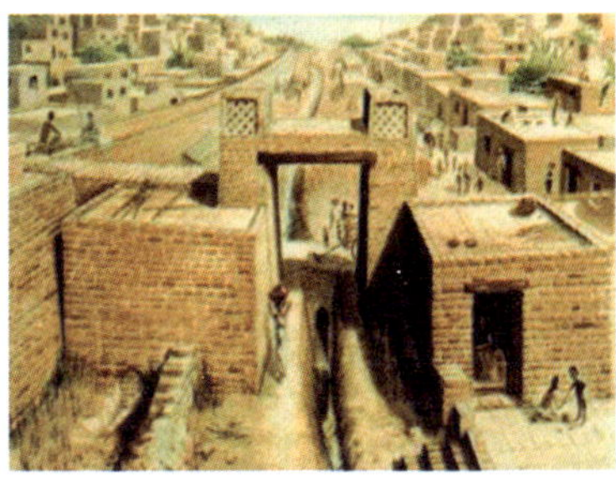

*The Indus Valley Civilization*

Since then, the world has seen the advent

of hundreds of languages and many mediums of communication. Today, a person sitting in one corner of the world can get in touch with a person in the opposite corner of the world within moments. The advancement in science and technology has made the process of communication very easy.

## Quick Facts

- **Early modern communication took place in three main modes: spoken words, manuscript writing, especially letters and the print. Oral communication was the oldest of these three.**
- **Beginning from the Renaissance, writing developed as an important form of personal expression, particularly among the educated and the upper classes.**
- **Posts and Telegraphs, Telephone, Fax, Pagers, E-mail and Chatting (through Internet) are some of the modern means of communication.**
- **Radio and Television, Newspapers and Cinema are some of the modern means of mass communication in the present world.**

Chapter - 10

# TYPES OF COMMUNICATIONS

Communication means to contact others and to send and receive messages. We express ourselves through speaking, writing and indicating.

Communication through speech is called *verbal communication*.

Communication through writing and indicating is called *non-verbal communication*.

The different mediums through which we send our messages are called communication systems.

**The two types of communication systems are:**

- Personal Communication
- Mass Communication

## Personal Communication

The process through which we send and receive messages and information to and from an individual is called personal communication.

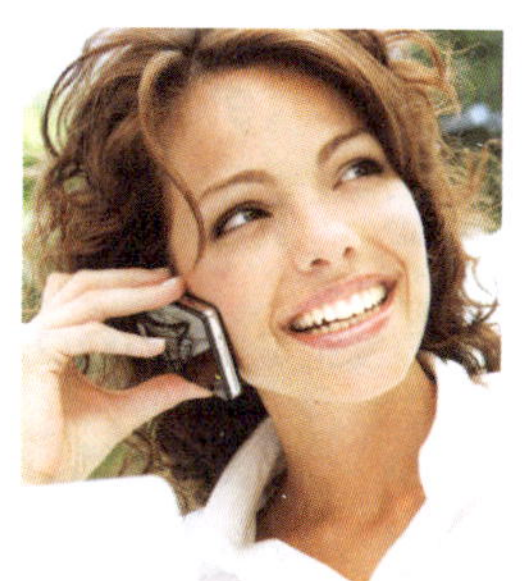

For example, writing a letter to your friend or speaking to your relative on a phone. Also, e-mailing and chatting on Internet with a person is a part of personal communication.

Following mediums are used in personal communication:

- Post
- Telegraph
- Telephone
- E-mail and Internet

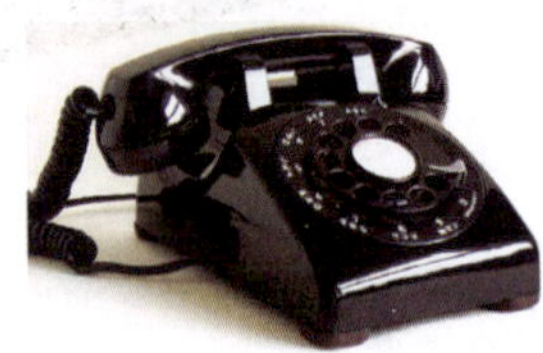

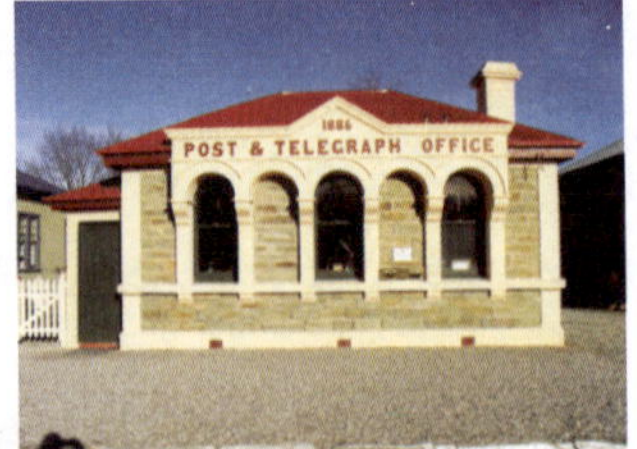


Advantages of Personal Communication:

- We can communicate directly with the person we want to communicate.
- It gives us flexibility of time and place. We can talk on phone or mobile from anywhere.
- It gives us privacy.

## Mass Communication

The process through which we send messages and information to a large group of people (or masses) is called mass communication. It doesn't give information to one person, but to the community at large.

For example, a newsreader reading news on radio and television.

The following mediums are used in mass communication:

- Newspapers and Magazines
- Radio
- Television
- Internet

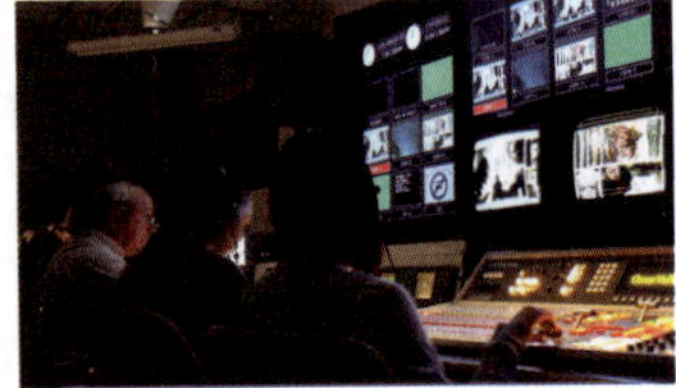

*Means of Mass Communication*

**Mass communication is divided into:**

- **Print Communication** – Newspapers, magazines, leaflets, pamphlets, brochures, etc.

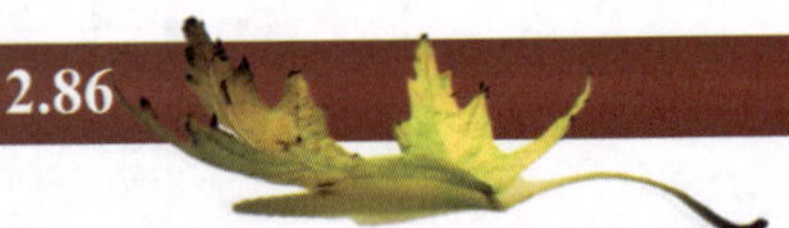

- **Electronic Communication** – Radio, Television and Internet.

**Advantages of Mass Communication:**

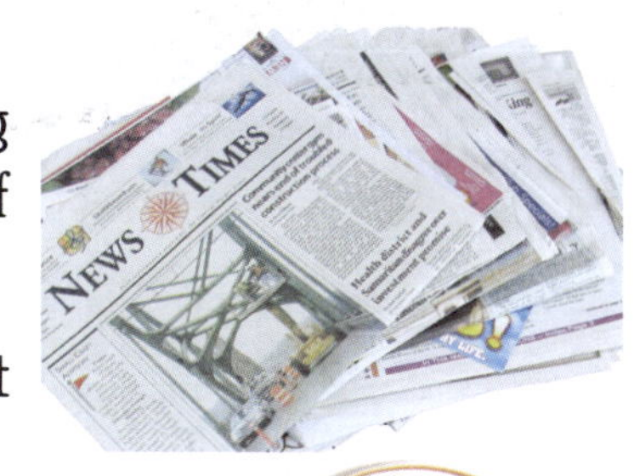


- They are very useful for sending information to a very large group of people.
- Everyone gets the information almost at the same time.

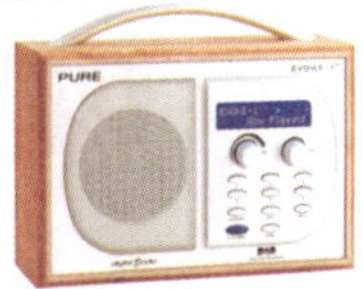

- Very low cost as compared to the personal means of communication.

## Quick Facts

- **Based on the style and purpose of communication, there can be two broad categories: Formal and Informal Communication, that have their own set of characteristic features.**
- **Formal Communication includes all the instances where communication has to occur in a set formal format. Typically, this can include all sorts of business or corporate communication.**
- **Informal Communication includes instances of free and unrestrained conversation between people who share a casual rapport with each other, such as friends, family members.**
- **Even though the whole process of communication may seem so simple, the effectiveness of each type depends to a great extent on certain internal and external environmental factors and also on the communicator's ability to send, receive, decode and send a response.**

Chapter - 11

# POST AND TELEGRAPH

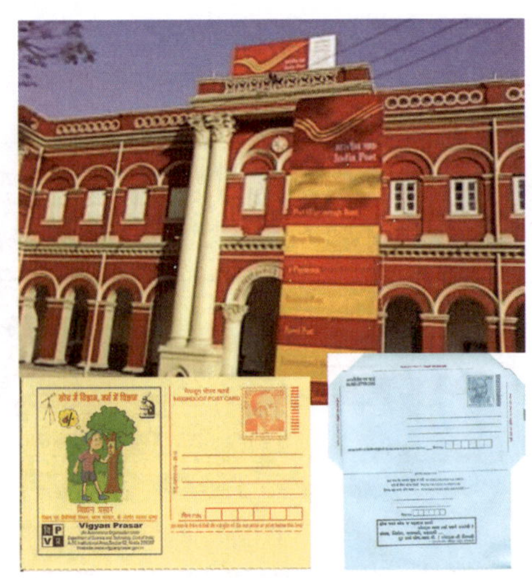


Post and Telegraph are very important means of personal communication.

Before the advent of modern means of communications like telephone, radio, television and internet, letters and other means of postal communications were the only significant media of personal communication.

## Do You Know?

The **Indian Post Office** was set up in the year **1854**.

### How does a postal system work?

The process of postal system starts as soon as you dispatch your properly addressed letter (including the postal/pin/zip code) in a letter box. The letters and posts from these public letter boxes get collected into a post office, where they are sorted into different stacks according to their post codes. Then these posts and letters are dispatched to different regions. Once your letter reaches to the post office of the specified office, a postman collects it and delivers it in your correspondent's address.

## Postal Service in India

In India, the Department of Posts is a government-operated postal service. The Indian Postal Service is the most widely used postal service in the world. There are around 1,55,333 post offices in our country.

The Indian Postal Service was first established under the East India Company, during the British rule, under the name, Company Mail in 1688. The possession of the postal service was given to the Indian Post Office in the year 1854.

## Stamps

The *adhesive stamps* were first introduced on October 1, 1854 in India. These were the first in Asia.

**Types of Postal Services**

**International Registered Post –** It is sent when the sender wishes to have a receipt of the mail from the receiver.

**Speed Post –** It is sent when the sender wants the mail to reach the next day, anywhere in the country.

**Parcels –** It is used for sending parcels upto 35 kg anywhere in the country.

## Quick Facts

- Post or Postal Codes are specific codes given to each area of a city/town in every region of a country. A post code makes it easier for your post to reach the desired place conveniently and on time.
- The highest post office of the world is at the height of about 15,500 feet in Hikkim, Himachal Pradesh.
- In 2011, the Indian Postal Service inaugurated a floating post office in the Dal Lake, Srinagar, Jammu & Kashmir.
- At the time of independence of India, there were about 23,344 post offices, which were primarily in urban areas.
- As of March 31, 2011, the Indian Postal Service has been recorded to have 154,866 post offices, of which 139,040 (89.78%) are in rural areas and around15,826 (10.22%)in urban areas. It has about 25,464 departmental POs and 129,402 ED BPOs.
- The U.S. Postal Service is the core of the trillion dollar mailing industry which employs more than 8 million people.

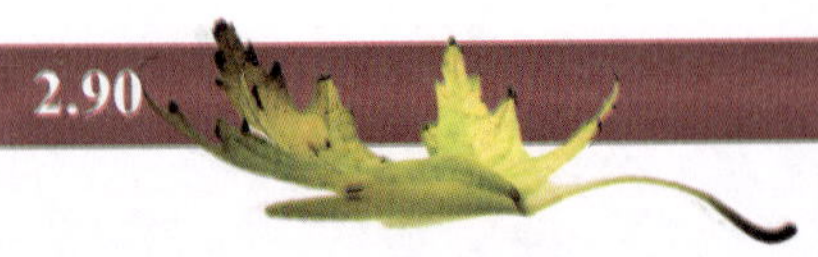

# Chapter - 12

# TELEPHONE

The word, 'telephone' is made up of two words, *tele* meaning 'distance' and *phonetics* meaning sound. Thus, Telephone means *sound from a distance*.

## How Does a Telephone Work?

**Process:** A telephone consists of a microphone which converts sound waves into electric current and sends it through a telephone network to another phone. The earphone or speaker in the receiving phone converts this electric signal back into sound wave.

## Do You Know?

**Alexander Graham Bell** was the first person to invent a telephone in the year **1876**.

## Advent of Telephones

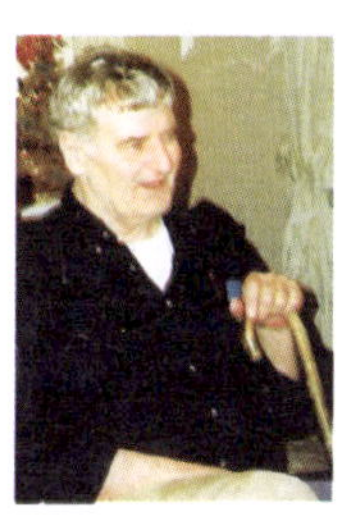

In the beginning, there was only one kind of telephone – *a fixed cable handset with a receiver and a body* with a dial pad. It is known as 'Landline' today. As the technology progressed, a new kind of phone came into being – a cordless phone.

**George Sweigert**, in **1966**, invented the **cordless phone** – a portable phone without a cable. It consisted of a handset with speaker/receiver and a base station. This phone could be carried around within a specified range of the base station. This provided tremendous flexibility to the user. The only drawback was that it needed to be plugged into the base for charging.

Then in **1973**, **Dr. Martin Cooper** of **Motorola** came out with the first mobile phone of the history. This is hailed as one of the biggest resolution in the field of telecommunication. Today, almost every person carries a mobile phone.

## Telephone Services in India

Today, there are around *33.19 million landline phones in India. India is world's second largest mobile phone using nation with over 881 million users, in 2011*. Also, it is the world's third largest internet using nation with over 121 million users, in 2011.

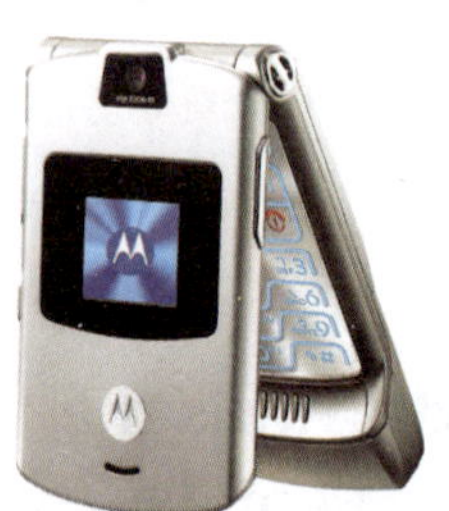

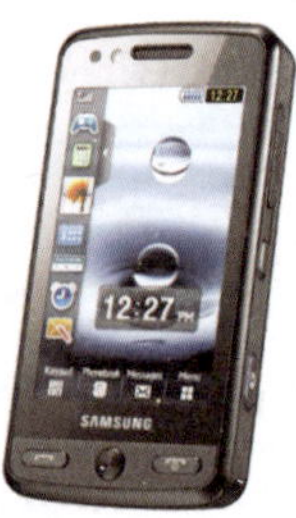

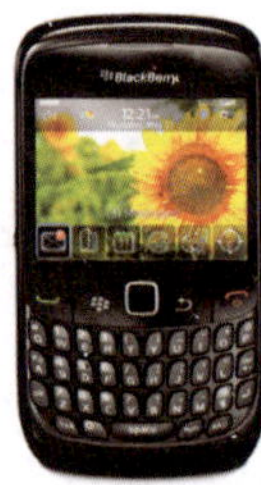

Today with the arrival of smart phones, people have got most of the telecommunication features in their handset. A smart phone has features like internet surfing, e-mailing, chat, message texting, etc.

## Advantages of Telephone:

- It is the easiest mode of personal communication today.
- With the advent of mobile phones, telecommunications have left behind all the other modes of communication as the most frequently used communication medium.

### Quick Facts

- **The first cellular phone network was established in the United States in the year 1983.**
- **Our telephone is made up of 201 parts, every one of which had to be planned, produced and assembled with an unusual degree of accuracy.**
- **As a tribute to Alexander Graham Bell when he died in 1922, all the telephones stopped ringing for one full minute.**
- **The great author and writer, Mark Twain was one of the first to have a phone in his home.**
- **Alexander Graham Bell thought the phone should be answered with "Hoy, Hoy" instead of "Hello".**
- **In 1956 the first transatlantic telephone cable was placed on the ocean floor and rests as deep as 12,000 feet! It runs from Newfoundland, Canada to Scotland!**
- **There are about 149,084,370 telephone lines in the world and thousands more are being added every day.**

Chapter - 13

# NEWSPAPERS AND MAGAZINES

Newspapers were the earliest means of mass communication. Newspapers and magazines come under the *print communication*.

## Newspapers

Around the world, newspapers are the most sought after means of communication for all the information regarding national events, political news, sports, science, technology, economics, business and trade, current affairs.

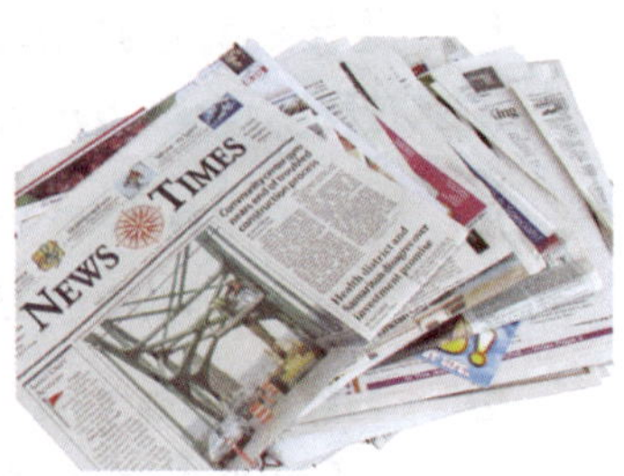


**Newspapers are divided into:**

- **National Dailies:** Newspapers which are circulated throughout the country are called national dailies. For example, *Hindustan Times, The Times of India, Indian Express* in English and *Hindustan, Navbharat Times, Dainik Bhaskar* in Hindi.
- **Regional Newspapers:** Newspapers which are circulated within a specific region are called regional newspapers. For example, *The Hindu* in south India, *Dainik Jagran* in north India.

- **Tabloids:** Newspapers which are not circulated in the morning, but are circulated during the noon or evening are called tabloids. For example, *Mail Today, Afternoon Despatch & Courier, Mid Day*, etc.

*The Bengal Gazette was the first newspaper to be published in India*, in the year, 1780, in Calcutta (Kolkata).

## Do You Know?

*By the year, 2007, there were around 6580 daily newspapers* being published across the world.

## Magazines

Apart from newspapers, magazines constitute a large share of the print communication. In India, around *75 popular magazines are published every year*. Magazines are generally based on the following subjects:

- Current affairs
- Politics
- Business
- Economics
- Science and technology
- Sports
- Entertainment
- Lifestyle

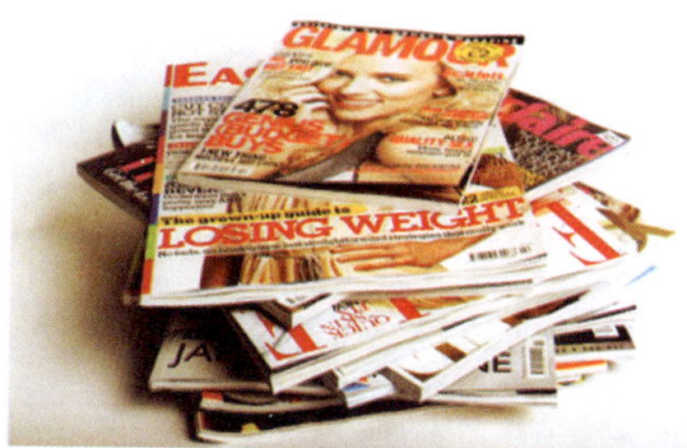


*Magazines*

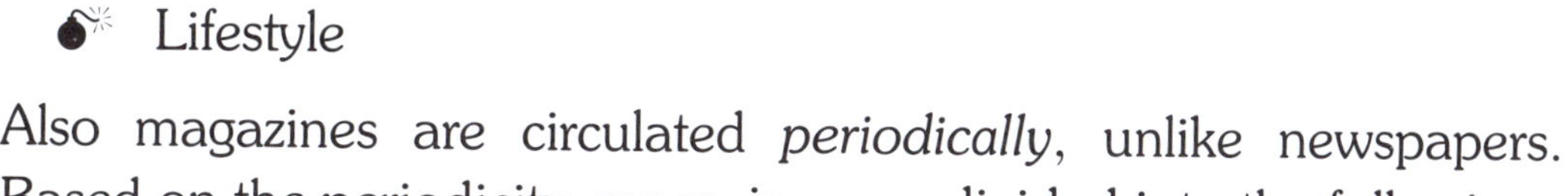

Also magazines are circulated *periodically*, unlike newspapers. Based on the periodicity, magazines are divided into the following:

- Weekly – Published every week
- Fortnightly – Published every 15 days
- Monthly – Published every month
- Quarterly – Published every three months
- Annually – Published once a year

**Advantages of Newspapers and Magazines:**

- They have a longer shelf life than television or radio. It means that people can keep their copy of newspaper/magazine with them and read or refer it again whenever they want to.
- They have greater reach in the local difficult terrain where radio or television signals don't reach.

## Quick Facts

- **The newspaper began its roots as early as Julius Caesar times. During that time, it was regarded as those scrolls read in front of the public to inform them of important happenings and events. Its first recorded account was as early as 59 B.C. and the name of the first newspaper was Acta Diurna.**
- **The Gentleman's Magazine, first published in 1731, in London, is considered to have been the first general-interest magazine. Edward Cave, who edited The Gentleman's Magazine under the pen name, 'Sylvanus Urban', was the first to use the term, 'magazine', on the analogy of a military storehouse of varied material, ultimately derived from the Arabic-makhazin ('storehouses') by way of the French language. The oldest consumer magazine still in print is The Scots Magazine, which was first published in 1739.**

# RADIO

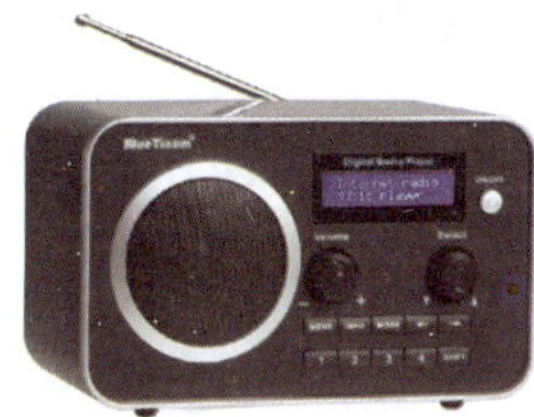
A Modern Radio

Radio is the most basic as well as one of the earliest means of electronic communication. It is the *first wireless communication system in the world*.

## How Does a Radio Transmission Work?

Radio transmission uses the concept of electromagnetic waves to send and receive information.

**Process:** The *sound energy is converted into electrical energy*. This electrical energy is sent to a transmitter which converts this electric current into electromagnetic waves. These electromagnetic waves are then transmitted into the atmosphere. A radio set acts as a receiver. The *antenna* in a radio set catches the electromagnetic waves. These waves are then turned into electric current. This electric current is then converted into sound energy which we can hear in the form of *music*, *news*.

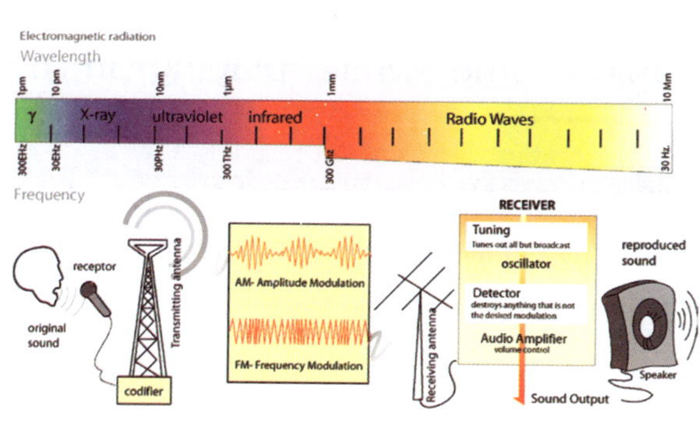

Electromagnetic Radiation

## Do You Know?

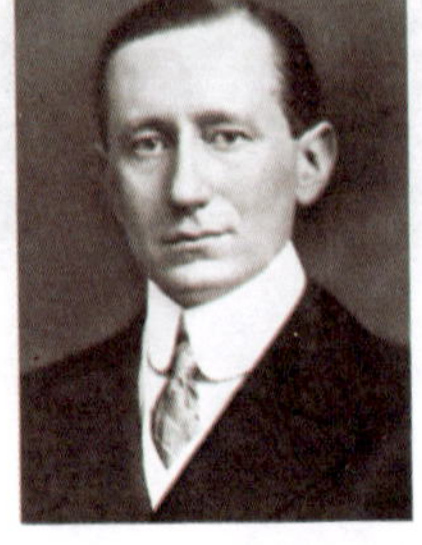

**Guglielmo Marconi** of Italy was the first to send and receive the first radio signals in **1895**.

**A radio runs on the following band widths:**

- **AM** – Amplitude Modulation
- **FM** – Frequency Modulation

Most of the private radio stations are based on FM.

## Radio Broadcasting in India

The *first radio broadcast in India took place on July 23, 1927*.

It was broadcasted by the *Indian Broadcasting Company (IBC)* which inaugurated its *first radio station in Bombay (Mumbai)*.

Bombay (Mumbai), Calcutta (Kolkata), Madras (Chennai) and Bangalore (Bengaluru) were the first few cities to have radio stations in the country.

Today, there are on an average 10 radio stations (mostly FM) in important cities of the country. These stations include private as well as public radio stations.

### Advantages of Radio for Mass Communication

- Radio is a universal medium and can be used at any time.
- It does not have to be viewed or read unlike other mediums. Therefore, it saves people's time while playing in the background.
- People can give their feedback on the content of the program by 'phoning' the radio stations, or by sending sms through their mobiles, by sending e-mails through the Internet.
- Information broadcast through radio can even be useful for the illiterate people.

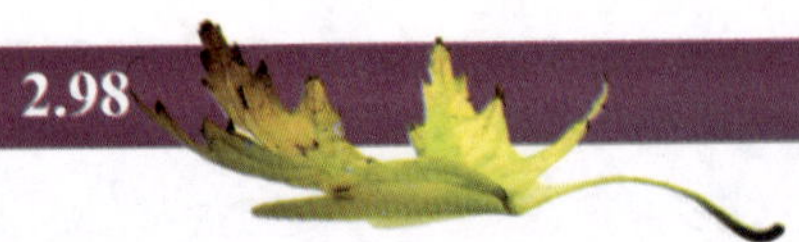

## Quick Facts

- Radio frequencies are between 300 GHz to 3 Hz.
- The Radio waves travel at a speed of about 186,000 miles per second, and were discovered in 1865 by James Clerk Maxwell.
- The All India Radio (AIR) is the government broadcasting body in India.
- FM broadcasting is preferred over AM broadcasting because FM transmissions are not disturbed by static interference. Also, FM transmissions have better sound quality.
- The Radio waves are considered to be Electromagnetic Radiations.
- An Amplitude Modulation (AM) wave is considered to be as long as a football field.
- Edwin Howard Armstrong, a genius by birth invented the Frequency Modulation (FM) band.

# Chapter - 15

# TELEVISION

*Television is the most important medium of electronic communication.*The term, 'Television' is made up of the Greek word, *tele* which means 'far' and the Latin word, *visio* which means 'sight'. Thus, television means 'seeing from the distance'.

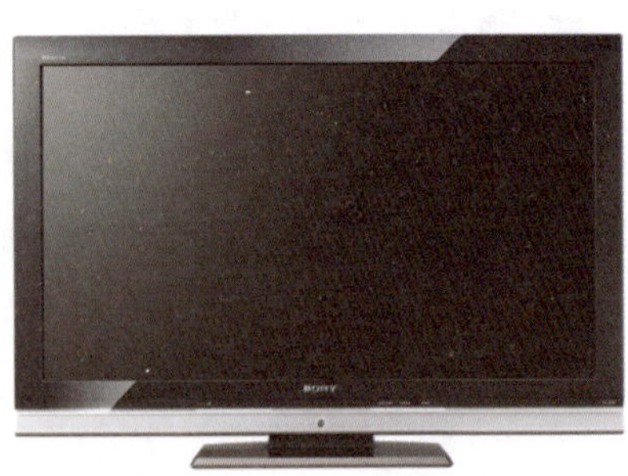

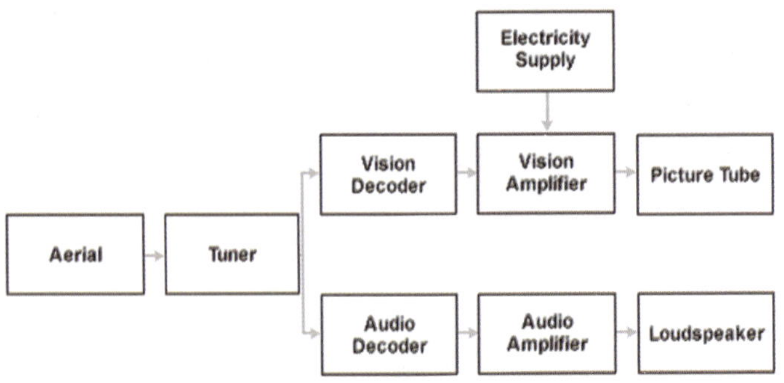


A television is a telecommunication medium which receives and displays moving images along with the sounds.

## How Does a Television Work?

**Process:** The data (audio-video) is converted into electric signal. This electric signal is then transmitted through a transmitter into the atmosphere. These signals are then received by an antenna which converts them back into audio and video data. This data is then seen and heard on the television screen and speakers.

## Do You Know?

**Philo Farnsworth** of Great Britain transmitted the television image in **1927**.

## Television in India

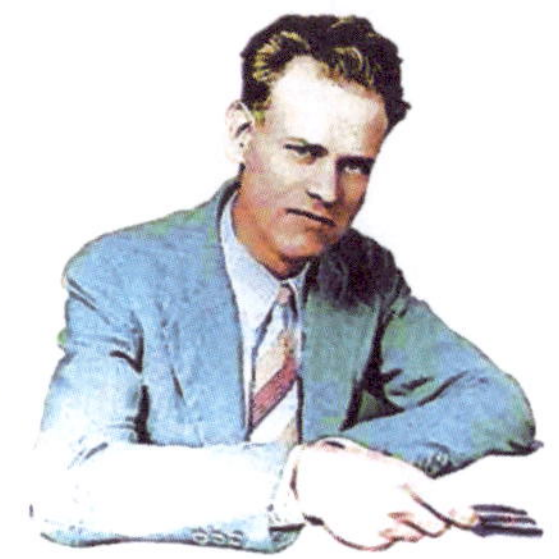

*Philo Farnsworth*

Television is one of the main media of information as well as entertainment for people. Earlier, there were only two channels on Indian television, i.e., DD National and DD Metro. But today, there is a number of private channels like Star, Zee, Sony, etc.

There are all kinds of program broadcasted on television like news, entertainment, sports shows, quiz shows, fiction serials, etc.

## Advantages of Television:

- Very useful for illiterate people who can take advantage of the fact that it is an audio-visual medium.
- People get latest information and news because of instantaneous transmission services.
- It plays an important part in educating the people on several important issues. Being a visual medium, it has a greater impact on people's thinking.

## Quick Facts

- In 1938, the television broadcasts were, for the first time, able to be taped and edited. Prior to that, only live transmission was possible.
- India is the third largest television viewing nation in the world, following China and the United State (US) the US, being the first.
- National telecasts were introduced in India in the year 1982.
- In 1982, the coloured television sets came into the Indian market.
- In the year 1926, J.L. Baird first displayed television which had only 30 lines and gave coarse image. Currently the digital signal of the television sends pictures with 1080 lines.
- A 103-inch plasma TV from Panasonic is the largest plasma TV currently available in the market, costing approximately around $70,000.

# THE INTERNET

*Internet is the latest and most convenient medium of mass communication*. The Internet is a worldwide system of interconnected computer networks that uses certain guidelines called the *Internet Protocols* to give information to people across the globe.

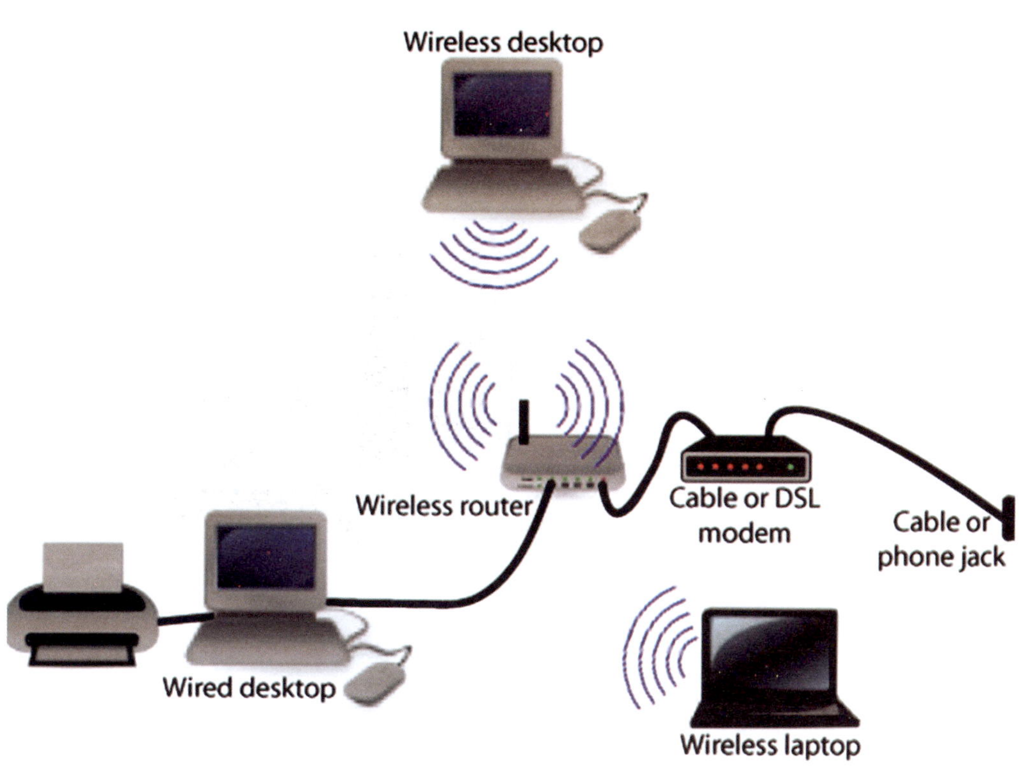

## How Does the Internet Work?

**Process:** The Internet is a huge structure of interconnected computer networks. These networks have a number of computers under them. In a network, computers are connected to a server. A server is a system which receives the information from the *router*. A router is the link between the network and the Internet. This router gathers information from communication mediums like *telephone lines, satellites, fibre-optic cables*, etc.

## Do You Know?

An Internet is a result of the research conducted by the *United States of America in 1960, for the development of computer networks.*

## Internet in India

*India is the world's fourth largest Internet using nation with over 121 million users in 2011*. In the year, **1995**, the **Videsh Sanchar Nigam Ltd. (VSNL)** introduced the Internet in India. By 2005, around 40 million people in the country were regular users of the Internet.

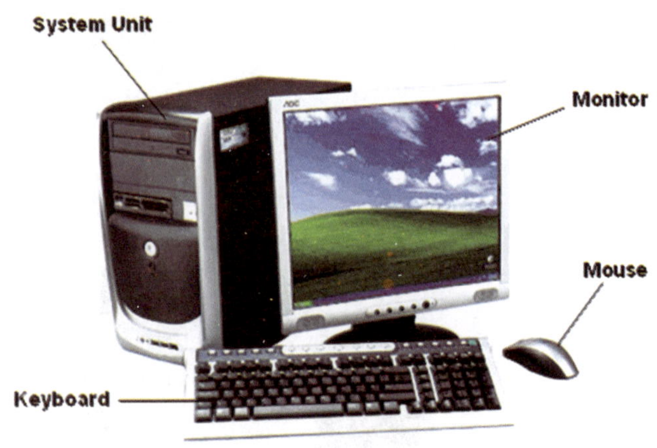


Today, there are around *180 Internet service providing companies in the country*, such as MTNL, VSNL, Airtel, Aircel, Sify, Reliance, Tata.

## Advantages of the Internet:

- It allows greater flexibility in working hours.
- It can be accessed by a number of mediums like mobile, data cards. It doesn't require a wired network.
- You can have access to almost any information in the world.
- It gives you information, entertainment, latest news, trading platform, shopping platform, e-banking, and many such services.
- *E-mail, chats and social networking* are good platforms for giving out information and being in touch with a large number of people.

## Quick Facts

- **The World Wide Web (WWW) came into existence in the year 1994.**
- **An Internet service provider is a company which operates the Internet on various networks like the Local Area Network (LAN) and the World Area Network (WAN).**
- **The Internet grew at a much faster pace than the Radio and TV as it reached 50 million users in just 5 years, whereas the Radio and TV took 38 and 13 years respectively to reach this target. Out of this, 35.6 percent of Internet users are Asian.**
- **The first webcam was deployed at the Cambridge University computer lab with the sole purpose to monitor a particular coffee maker and hence, avoid wasted trips to an empty pot.**

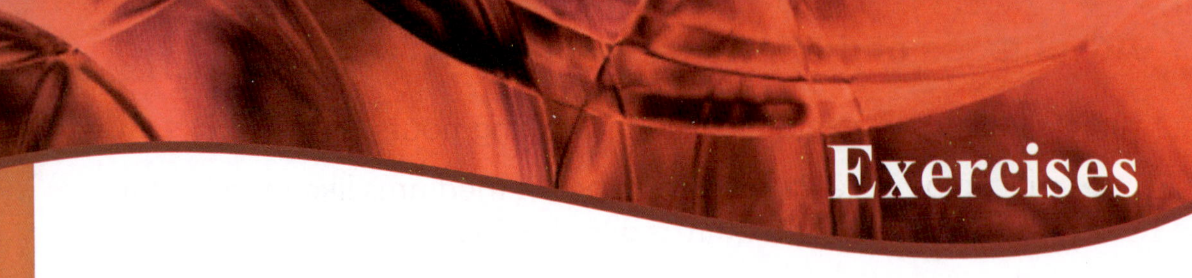

# Exercises

## I. Answer the following questions.

Q.1. What do you understand by the term, 'Transportation'?

Q.2. Name some common means of Transport used particularly in India.

Q.3. What is Fuel? What are the different types of fuels used in various vehicles?

Q.4. Can you name some major means of ancient transportation?

Q.5. When did roads and bridges come into existence?

Q.6. When did the invention of automobile take place?

## II. Fill in the blanks with suitable words.

1. The word, 'car' has been derived from the ____________ word, *carrus* which means 'wheeled vehicle'.
2. In the year, 1903 ___________ brothers, ____________ and ______________ demonstrated the first ever airplane with a propeller.
3. By ______________, most of the railway networks in the world had started ________________.
4. The first steam engine was invented by ____________.
5. There are mainly three types of _____________.

## III. Match the two columns correctly.

| | A | B |
|---|---|---|
| 1. | The stone-paved roads were first built in | concrete, asphatt, stone and gravel. |
| 2. | Modern roads are generally made up of | third largest road network in the world. |
| 3. | India has the | Mesopotamia. |
| 4. | There are basically three types of rails | Broad gauge, Metre gauge and the narrow gauge. |
| 5. | A harbour is a place | where ships, boats and ferries take shelter. |

## IV. Multiple Choice Questions (MCQs)

1. Jebel Ali in Dubai is the ___________.

   (a) smallest artificially created harbour.

   (b) largest artificially created harbour.

   (c) not an artificially created harbour.

   (d) natural harbour.

2. Goa, Kochi, Panjim, Pondicherry and Mangalore are some of the ___________.

   (a) well-known harbours in India.

   (b) well-known ports in India.

   (c) artificial harbours in India.

   (d) natural harbour in India.

3. Concorde is a/an ______________ aircraft.

(a) infrasonic (b) supersonic

(c) ultrasonic (d) none of these

4. A submarine is a watercraft which moves ____________.

(a) above the surface of water

(b) along the surface of water

(c) below the surface of water

(d) on both land and water

5. The Bullet Train is also known as ____________.

(a) Min Kansen (b) Jim Kansen

(c) Rim Kansen (d) Shin Kansen

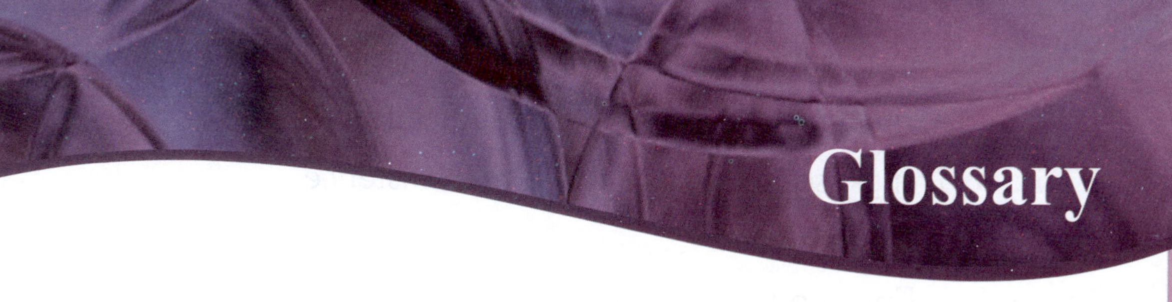

# Glossary

**Pedalling:** To move pedals of a bicycle and ride it

**Rickshaws:** A small, light vehicle used to carry passengers

**Paved:** To prepare or make easier

**Mast:** A structure rising above the hull/upper part of a ship or a boat

**Palanquin:** A covered litter, formerly used in India, carried on the shoulders of four men

**Emission:** Radiation

**Carriages:** A wheeled vehicle for carrying people drawn by horses

**Commercial:** Suitable or fit for a wide, popular market

**Locomotive:** A self-propelled, vehicular engine powered by steam, diesel/electricity

**Conveyance:** The process of taking somebody/something from one place to another

**Sleigh:** Another name for sledge, i.e., a vehicle drawn by horses or dogs

**Convenient:** Easy, suitable, agreeable

**Revenue:** The income of a government from taxation, excise duties, customs

**Purview:** Range of operation, authority

**Concrete:** An artificial stone like material

**Approve:** To consent or agree to

**Freight:** Transportation of goods by ships, planes, trains or lorries

**Lifeline:** A vital line of access or communication

**Entities:** Things, something having a real existence

**Efficiency:** Competency

**Excessive:** Enormous, extravagant

**Alternative:** A possibility of choice, either of such choices

**Frequency:** Regularity, periodicity, how often

**Hovercraft:** A vehicle that travels just above the surface of water or land, held up by air being forced downwards

**Transit:** An act of passing across or through

**Consumption:** Utilisation, depletion

**Amplifier:** An electronic device used to increase the strength of sound or radio signal

**Device:** Machine, instrument

**Electronic:** Concerned with or operated by devices in which electrons are conducted through a body

**Fluctuation:** Continual change from one point condition to another

**Transmission:** Transfer, passing of

**Impedes:** Blocks, thwarts, checks

**Insert:** To put in or between, introduce

**Indispensable:** Essential, absolutely necessary

**Broad casting:** To transmit or relay programmes on radio or television

**Modulation:** Variation, intonation, transition, inflection

**Feedback:** Response or reaction



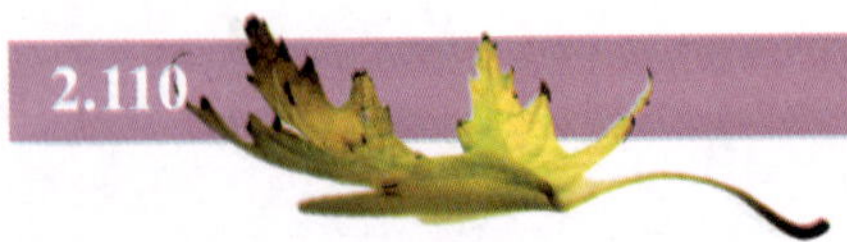

**Displays:** Shown or exhibits, unfolds

**Converts:** Transforms, to change, to alter

**Interconnected:** Interrelated, interlinked

**Protocol:** A set of rules that controls the way date is sent between computers

**Accessed:** Judged, verified, adjudged

# V&S OLYMPIAD GUIDE BOOK AND WORKBOOK SERIES (CLASSES 1-10)

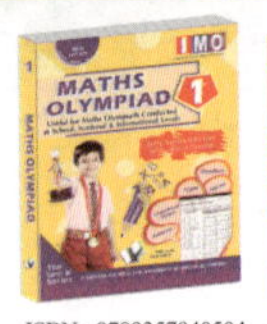
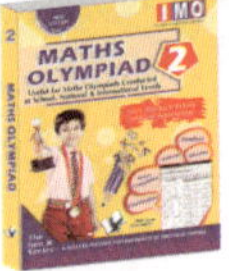
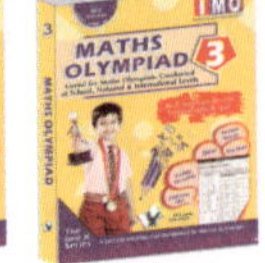
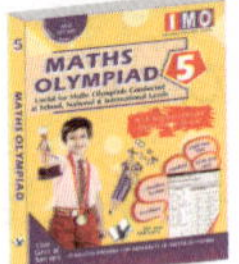
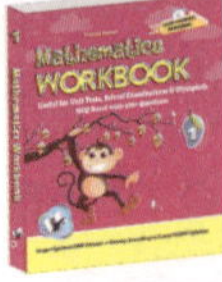
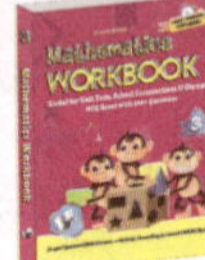
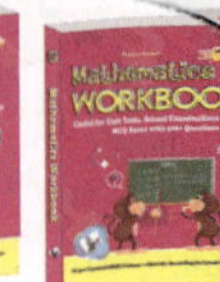

ISBN : 9789357940504 ISBN : 9789357940511 ISBN : 9789357940528 ISBN : 9789357940535 ISBN : 9789357940542

ISBN : 9789357942447 ISBN : 9789357942454 ISBN : 9789357942461 ISBN : 9789357942478 ISBN : 97893579424

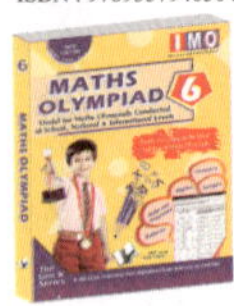
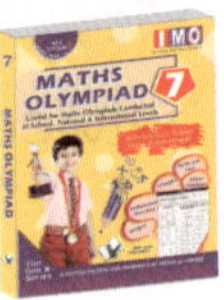
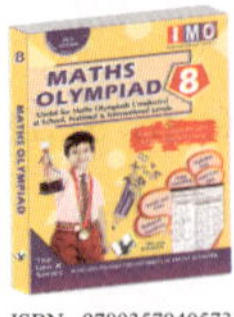
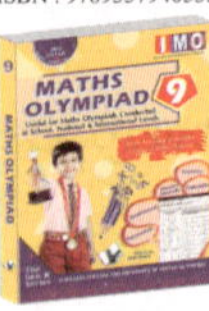
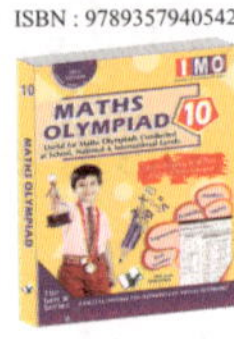
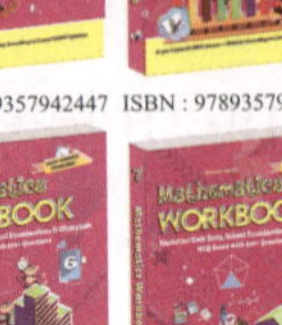
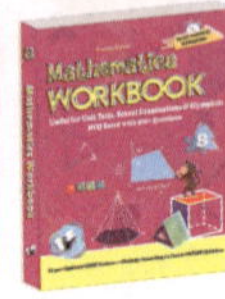
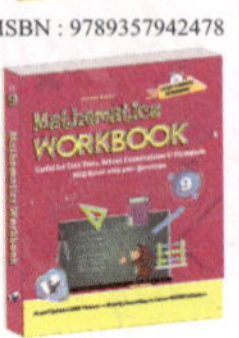
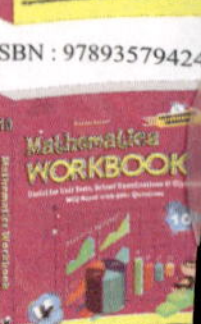

ISBN : 9789357940559 ISBN : 9789357940566 ISBN : 9789357940573 ISBN : 9789357940580 ISBN : 9789357940597

ISBN : 9789357942492 ISBN : 9789357942508 ISBN : 9789357942515 ISBN : 9789357942522 ISBN : 97893579425

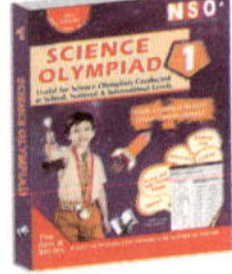
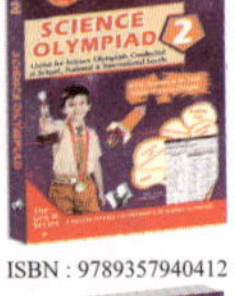
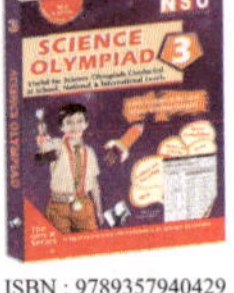
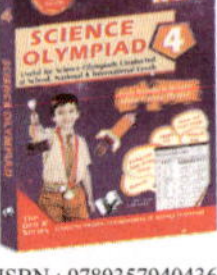
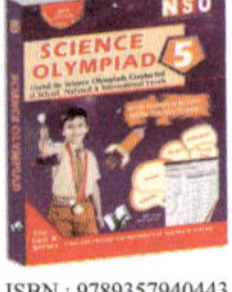
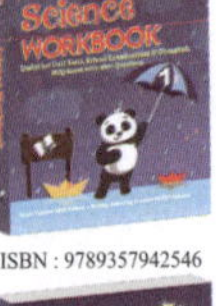
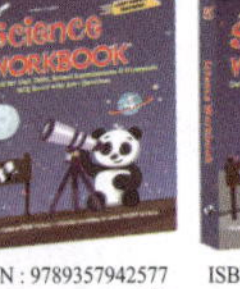

ISBN : 9789357940405 ISBN : 9789357940412 ISBN : 9789357940429 ISBN : 9789357940436 ISBN : 9789357940443

ISBN : 9789357942546 ISBN : 9789357942553 ISBN : 9789357942560 ISBN : 9789357942577 ISBN : 97893579425

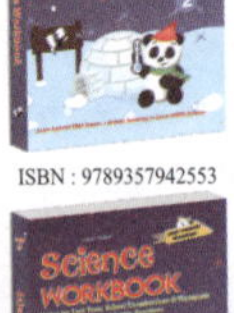
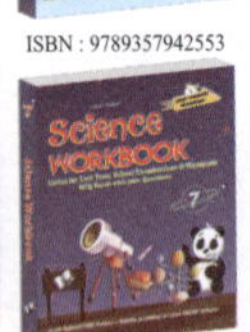
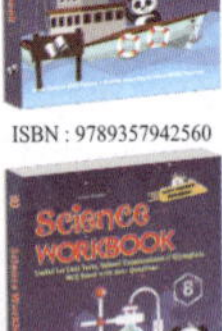
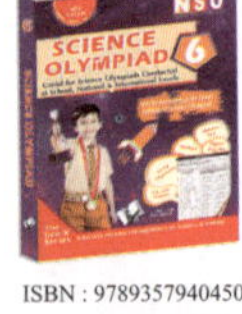
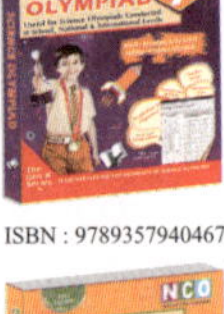

ISBN : 9789357940450 ISBN : 9789357940467 ISBN : 9789357940474 ISBN : 9789357940481 ISBN : 9789357940498

ISBN : 9789357942591 ISBN : 9789357942607 ISBN : 9789357942614 ISBN : 9789357942621 ISBN : 978935794

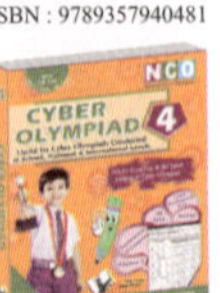
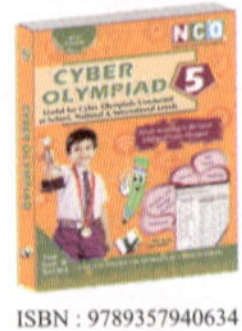
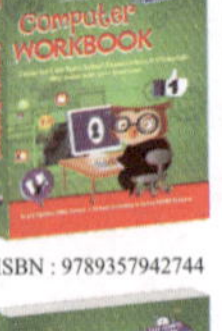
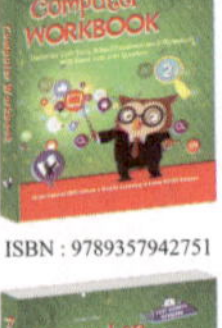
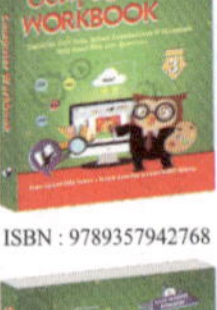
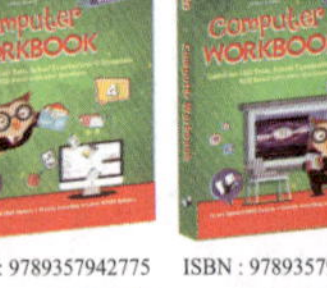

ISBN : 9789357942102 ISBN : 9789357940603 ISBN : 9789357940610 ISBN : 9789357940627 ISBN : 9789357940634

ISBN : 9789357942744 ISBN : 9789357942751 ISBN : 9789357942768 ISBN : 9789357942775 ISBN : 978935794

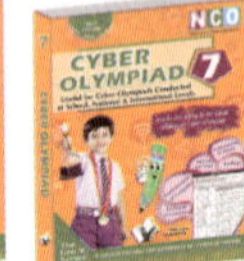
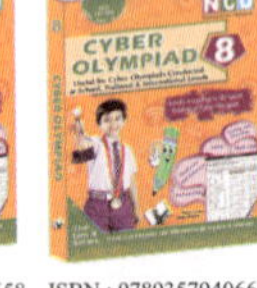
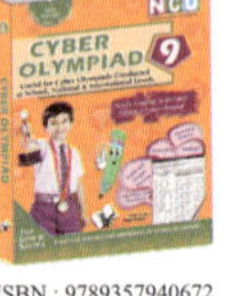
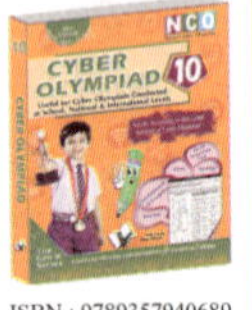
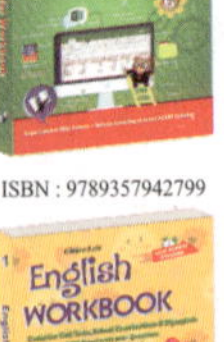

ISBN : 9789357940641 ISBN : 9789357940658 ISBN : 9789357940665 ISBN : 9789357940672 ISBN : 9789357940689

ISBN : 9789357942799 ISBN : 9789357942805 ISBN : 9789357942812 ISBN : 9789357942829 ISBN : 978935794

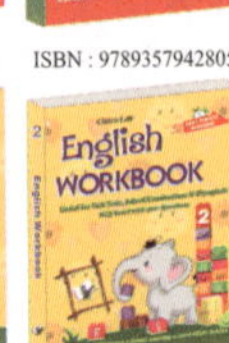
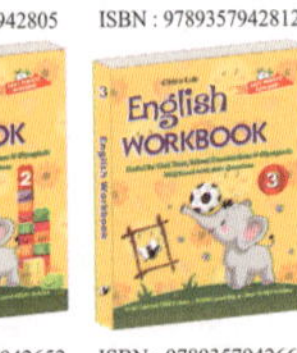
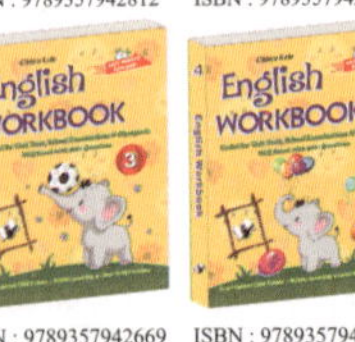
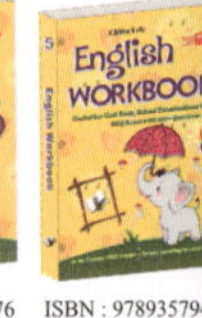

ISBN : 9789357940696 ISBN : 9789357940702 ISBN : 9789357940719 ISBN : 9789357940726 ISBN : 9789357940733

ISBN : 9789357942645 ISBN : 9789357942652 ISBN : 9789357942669 ISBN : 9789357942676 ISBN : 97893579

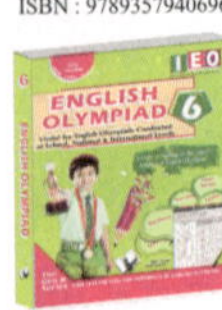
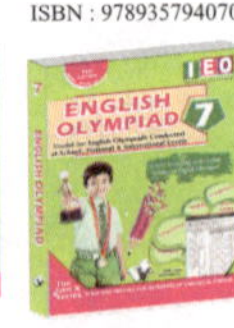
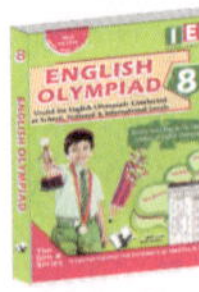
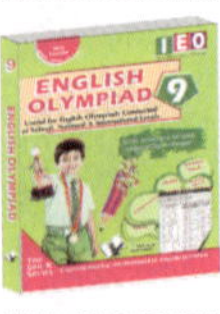
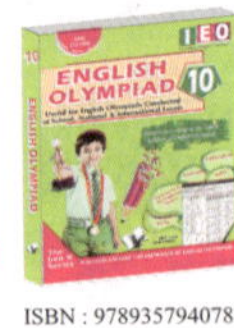

ISBN : 9789357940740 ISBN : 9789357940757 ISBN : 9789357940764 ISBN : 9789357940771 ISBN : 9789357940788

ISBN : 9789357942690 ISBN : 9789357942706 ISBN : 9789357942713 ISBN : 9789357942720 ISBN : 97893579

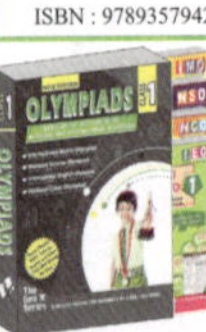

ISBN : 9789357942263 ISBN : 9789357942270 ISBN : 9789357942287 ISBN : 9789357942294 ISBN : 9789357942300

ISBN : 9789357942003 ISBN : 9789357942010 ISBN : 9789357942027 ISBN : 9789357942034 ISBN : 97893579

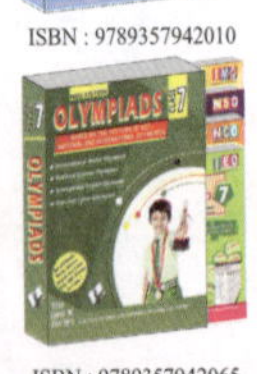
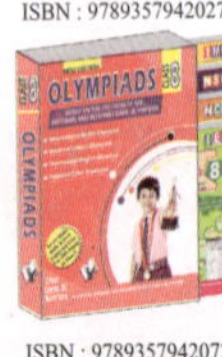
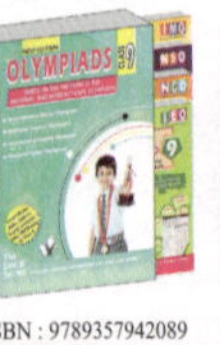
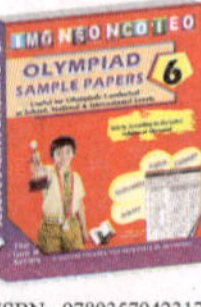
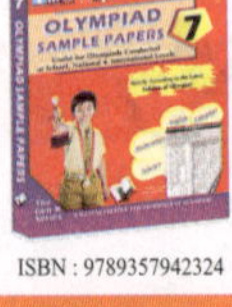
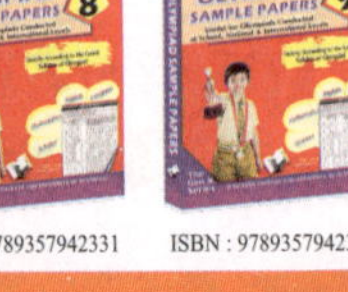
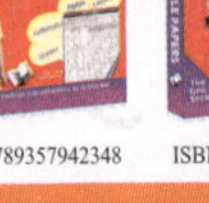

ISBN : 9789357942317 ISBN : 9789357942324 ISBN : 9789357942331 ISBN : 9789357942348 ISBN : 9789357942355

ISBN : 9789357942058 ISBN : 9789357942065 ISBN : 9789357942072 ISBN : 9789357942089 ISBN : 97893579

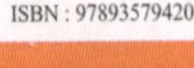
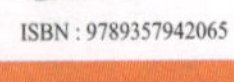